Praise for

ALZHEIMER'S TREATMENT
ALZHEIMER'S PREVENTION

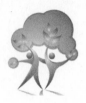

"A refreshingly optimistic perspective on prevention and treatment for a disease that has confronted many disappointing therapies. It is empowering for patients, caregivers, and clinicians."

—DANIEL A. COHEN, MD, MMSc
COGNITIVE NEUROLOGIST, E. VIRGINIA MEDICAL SCHOOL

"An outstanding review of the most current empirically validated strategies against AD that anyone can understand and apply. It's the 'How-to-Guide' for AD, written by one of the world's foremost authorities."

—CHRISTOPHER N. OCHNER, PhD
ASST. PROFESSOR OF CLINICAL PSYCHOLOGY,
COLUMBIA UNIVERSITY COLLEGE OF PHYSICIANS & SURGEONS

ALZHEIMER'S TREATMENT

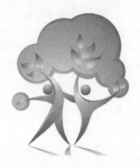

ALZHEIMER'S PREVENTION

A PATIENT AND FAMILY GUIDE

Thirty Questions Answered by Alzheimer's Expert

Richard S. Isaacson, M.D.

Associate Professor of Clinical Neurology
University of Miami—Miller School of Medicine

Published by AD Education Consultants, Inc.
Miami Beach, FL USA

For more information, visit: www.TheADplan.com

Follow us on Facebook! www.facebook.com/AlzheimersDisease

ISBN 978-0-9831869-7-7
Library of Congress Catalog Number 2011902501

Cover Design: Ciara Gaglio • www.cng-designs.com
Interior Design: Gary A. Rosenberg • www.garyarosenberg.com

*To my uncle Bob and cousins Cynthia,
Frankie, and Guy*

*To my dad's cousin Charlotte,
and her devoted husband, Phil*

To 'Grandpa' Artie, and 'Grandma' Sue

*And to my patients
and their amazing caregivers: I admire you.*

Contents

Section 3. Preventing Alzheimer's

Author's Note

"What a party!" Not the typical words you would expect to find at the beginning of a book on the challenging topic of Alzheimer's disease (AD). But these are the words that come to mind when I think about my great uncle Bob, who was the first person in my life to be diagnosed with the disease. Uncle Bob was always happy, smiling, telling jokes, and was, by far, *always* the life of the party. Alzheimer's first robbed him of his short-term memory, and then later his ability to care for himself, but I won't let his disease cloud my own memories of what an incredible person he was to me.

In 1961, my great uncle Bob was painting a house in Brooklyn, New York, when he asked the woman who hired him, "Who is the pretty girl in that picture?" My grandmother Ruth proudly replied, "That's a picture of my darling daughter."

He asked my grandma if she would allow him to introduce her to his nephew. Several months later, my dad and mom met.

Uncle Bob not only introduced my mom and dad, but several years later he again had a profound effect on my life. When I was three years old at a pool party at my aunt Carol's house, I fell into the pool and disappeared under the water. While my cousin Jeff ran for help, both instinctively and immediately, my uncle Bob jumped in to save me. It goes without saying that for several reasons, I appreciate all he did to get (and keep) me here today!

Uncle Bob began suffering from Alzheimer's when I was just starting medical school. It was frustrating that even though medicine had come so far, at that time there were essentially no treatments for the disease. Several years later and just months after I completed my neurology training, another family member began exhibiting the signs of AD. These personal experiences have instilled in me the empathy and motivation to dedicate my professional career to combating this most challenging disease.

As a neurologist working in an academic setting (University of Miami Miller School of Medicine), I divide my time between three areas: patient care, research, and education. I teach medical students and neurology residents in the outpatient clinic and at the bedside at Jackson Memorial Hospital, the third-largest public hospital and third-largest teaching hospital in the United States. In addition, I have lectured to faculty and trainees in internal medicine, family medicine, psychiatry, and geriatrics at the University of Miami and at several other institutions. I have been invited to lecture on the topic of "Recent Advances in the Management of Alzheimer's disease" and "Prevention of Alzheimer's disease" all over the country. These lectures are attended by physicians in a variety of specialties, as well as nurses, nurse practitioners, physician assistants, and other members of the healthcare team.

I have found that regardless of whether I am speaking to a group of neurologists at a large academic medical center in the Northeast, or to a group of family practice physicians and nurse practitioners at a small private practice in the Midwest, there is a significant gap between potential treatments for Alzheimer's disease and what is actually recommended to patients.

This gap in treatment, as well as the personal experiences of my family members, patients, and close friends, prompted me to write this book.

—Richard S. Isaacson, M.D.

Acknowledgments

This book would not be possible without the help and collaboration of several individuals. My family played a significant role in my development as a person and as a physician. My dad was my biggest role model, and my brother my most significant career/life influence—I thank them both times a million for their love and eternal support. I would be remiss without thanking my mom (who makes the best chicken cutlets and Spanish chicken this side of the Mississippi), my sister Suzee, my sister and brother in-law Barbara and Mike, and my eight nieces and nephews.

A special thanks to: Drs. Chris Papasian and Daryl Thompson (for teaching me in the early days of medical school and guiding my path ever since); Drs. Clifford Saper, Michael Ronthal, and Louis Caplan (for mentorship, training, and for holding me to the highest standard of neurologic care);

Drs. Sacco, Pankau, Cohen, Zadikoff, Savitz, Rundek, Wright, Martinez, Dib, and Benatar; Ranee; J. LaRoe; the Helfner family; all my teachers/advisors at Commack High School for setting the foundation of my education and future (Jack McGrath, Bruce Leon, Sal Sinito, Ron Vale, and Dr. Doug and Susan Dreilinger); my best friends Justin, Chris, Reza, Brett, Dave, Brandon, Mike, Jared, Peter, Tonnie, Janie, Harold, Niko, Steve & Dr. Andy Tarulli; Cheryl Fawn for helpful insights into the importance of nutrition and adequate diet; H. Ron Davidson; Nataly Rubinstein; Dr. Marc Agronin; Ciara Gaglio for cover design; and last but not least, the N.Y. Yankees (for being the best sports franchise in the entire Universe!).

Introduction

ALZHEIMER'S DISEASE: AN UPDATE

Overview

Alzheimer's disease (AD) is a condition where an individual will progressively lose their memory and thinking skills. Oftentimes, patients will attribute these cognitive changes to a part of the normal aging process. However, as time goes on, short-term memory declines and the most common problems include loss of orientation (e.g., not knowing the date), difficulty with communication (e.g., finding the correct words to say), changes in behavior, and impaired judgment. Some examples of memory loss include continually losing things, like keys or a cell phone. Misplacing objects, forgetting appointments, and repeating the same things over and over again are also common symptoms, which may be related to memory and/or concentration. The first observable signs of AD may not actually be memory loss, but may instead be a depressed mood, a loss of interest in pleasurable activities, a change in personality, increasing anxiety, or even a change in sleep patterns. I am a strong advocate for early diagnosis, so it is advisable for patients to seek medical attention when symptoms first begin. A variety of specialists can be called upon to perform an evaluation, including primary care doctors (e.g., internist or family doctor), neurologists, geriatric psychiatrists, or geriatricians (who specialize in the care of patients aged 65 and over). As I have said time and time again, the earlier you diagnose, the earlier you can treat, and the earlier that you treat, the better the patient will do.

AD is the most common form of dementia, representing approximately two-thirds of all cases. The number-one risk factor for AD is advancing age. In fact, the most recent statistics show that one out of seven individuals aged 71 and over have dementia, and over 45% of individuals over the age of 85 have AD. According to the Alzheimer's Association 2011 statistics, there are over 5.4 million people in the United States with AD, and this number will nearly triple by the year 2050.

Treatment and Prevention

For the most part, the treatment and prevention strategies that are discussed in this book target specific biological abnormalities that occur in AD. Many of the prescription drugs used to treat AD aim to increase chemicals in the brain that help with memory and behavior. These chemicals have progressively become deficient in the brains of patients with AD. Other interventions to be discussed may aim to reduce inflammation in the brain (e.g., omega-3 fatty acids), improve blood flow (e.g., via optimizing control of abnormal blood pressure, blood sugar, and cholesterol), reduce the amount of detrimental protein deposits (e.g., exercise), or give the brain more "fuel" to function (e.g., medical food, very low-carbohydrate diet). AD is a very complex disease where scientists still do not entirely understand all of the intricacies. Some of the options discussed in this book have been shown to work or have the potential to work, but it is still unclear why. A great example here is exercise. For years clinicians recommended exercise for AD treatment and prevention because "it was good for you." Not a very scientific answer! In the past, physicians postulated that exercise increased blood flow to the brain or released chemicals into the bloodstream that improved memory and thinking skills, but proof was lacking. We now understand that regular exercise may help to increase blood flow to the brain and know more about which specific chemicals are released and how they make the brain work better.

Recent data has shown that regular exercise maintains cardiac function, and that alone correlates with larger brain volumes. Most recently, scientists have discovered that exercise reduces the pathologic protein in the AD brain called amyloid. A more detailed discussion of the neurobiology of AD and how each intervention for treatment and prevention "works" is beyond the scope of this book. Suffice it to say however that while we may not know exactly "how" some of these interventions work to improve symptoms or delay onset of AD, there is some clinical and/or scientific evidence of their effectiveness.

Diagnostic Criteria

While this book primarily focuses on the treatment and prevention strategies for AD, I want to briefly review the two most commonly used diagnostic criteria for this disease. For many years, physicians have used the "DSM-IV" criteria for diagnosing AD. DSM stands for the "Diagnostic and Statistical Manual of Mental Disorders" that was published by the American Psychiatric Association in 2000. In order to fulfill the criteria for AD, a patient needs to have the onset of memory problems plus one or more of the following:

1. problem with language or speaking skills (called "aphasia")

2. difficulty with performing movements or tasks, such as combing hair, brushing teeth, or driving (called "apraxia")

3. difficulty recognizing objects like a remote control to the television or a pencil (called "agnosia")

4. impaired judgment or thinking skills for everyday activities (called "executive function")

When these difficulties cause functional impairment enough to interfere with the normal activities of daily living, represent a decline from prior functioning, occur with a gradual onset and a slowly progressive course, and cannot be explained by any other non-brain disease (e.g., thyroid dysfunction, "pseudodementia" of depression), this would be most consistent with a diagnosis of dementia.

The earliest stages of AD are most often referred to as "mild Alzheimer's disease." As the disease progresses, physicians may then call the disease moderate AD, and as it continues to progress, severe AD. There is no clear consensus among physicians on when to use the terms *mild*, *moderate*, or *severe*. Some physicians will use results of cognitive testing, and others will conclude based on how the patient is functioning on an everyday basis.

In April 2011, new AD diagnostic criteria were published based on the recommendations of an expert panel convened by the National Institute on Aging and the Alzheimer's Association. These criteria include three "stages" of AD:

1. a diagnosis of dementia due to Alzheimer's disease

2. a diagnosis of mild cognitive impairment (MCI) due to Alzheimer's disease

3. "preclinical" Alzheimer's disease

These three classifications are helpful since they set the stage for future advances in AD by incorporating "biomarkers" in the diagnostic criteria. A biomarker is something that can be used to more accurately diagnose AD, like a blood test or a radiology study. At the time of publication of this book, there is no one single test available that can 100% surely diagnose AD, although in the future this may be possible. As an example, the earliest evidence of AD starts in the brain many years before we may observe clinical symptoms in patients.

Hopefully in the future, we will be able to perform a simple test (e.g., blood, spinal fluid, brain image) and then begin treatment many years before the onset of AD symptoms.

As mentioned in the new diagnostic criteria, mild cognitive impairment (also referred to as MCI) is commonly characterized by changes in thinking skills that have been identified by a physician, but these changes have not yet impacted the patient's activities of daily living. In my clinical experience, and now based on the new criteria, patients with MCI may most commonly have "pre-Alzheimer's," or prodromal AD (at risk for developing AD). Patients in this category may derive benefit from a variety of interventions that may be best suited for use early in the onset of memory loss. There are several ongoing scientific research trials that are currently studying this important area.

Diagnostic Testing

The most crucial aspect of AD diagnosis remains what doctors refer to as the "clinical history." A doctor will speak with the patient, family members, and friends to learn about the exact problems with memory. They will then ask specific questions and also perform a physical examination, asking questions to "test" memory and evaluate thinking skills. Afterward, doctors may order radiological studies (e.g., brain cat scan [CT] or magnetic resonance imaging [MRI]) and laboratory tests (e.g., blood work) to help determine the cause of their symptoms. When I lecture to healthcare providers across the country, I suggest specific recommendations that may help to improve their ability to arrive at an accurate diagnosis of AD. If ordering a brain MRI, requesting thin cuts through the hippocampus ("memory center" of the brain) or temporal lobes (e.g., MPRAGE sequence or epilepsy protocol, without contrast) may be a more "sensitive" way to detect abnormalities in that area.

When I order MRIs, I will ask the radiologist to assess for hippocampal atrophy (or "shrinkage" of the memory center of the brain), but it may be most optimal for an experienced Alzheimer's clinician to review the actual films, when possible. For each and every MRI ordered, I review the actual films myself. Most physicians will not feel comfortable with this, but certain AD specialists tend to agree with this approach. In my clinical practice, when a diagnosis remains unclear, I often consider detailed cognitive testing, called "neuropsychological testing." In addition to performing the actual testing, neuropsychologists often make excellent recommendations based on the specific cognitive deficits that are identified. I will also occasionally order another radiology study, called a PET scan (positron emission tomography), when the diagnosis remains in question.

Rise in Alzheimer's Cases

Many experts feel that the rise in AD cases is also due to a variety of factors other than the advancing age of our population, such as the improved ability to make an accurate diagnosis. Note that this would suggest that the incidence of AD had been much higher in previous years, but we are just now able to see this. With the advances of the medical field, doctors are now able to identify patients with AD in a variety of ways. We have learned a great deal about the brain and about brain aging, and can use the collected information to make a much more accurate diagnosis of Alzheimer's disease than in years past.

Other experts feel that based on the scientific evidence, one of the reasons that there has been an increase in the number of AD cases is the change in diet and nutrition patterns, particularly in the United States. As my colleague Dr. Christopher Ochner, a faculty member at Columbia University College of Physicians and Surgeons, has taught me, portion sizes, average meal intake, adult obesity, and childhood obesity are critical issues that need to be addressed and may certainly be related. Fast food on every corner, processed foods in every vending machine, and sugar, sugar, and more sugar added to just about anything and everything in arms reach. People are eating more fat and fewer fruits and vegetables than ever before. This "Western diet" has been extensively studied and results show that this type of diet is associated with a higher risk of developing AD (more on this later). By now, many of us understand that sugar is "bad" when it comes to the well-known condition of diabetes. But what is not yet fully understood are the long- and short-term effects of carbohydrates (e.g., sugar) on Alzheimer's disease.

Whatever the reason for the explosion of AD cases, in my clinical practice, I consider "anything and everything, as long as it is safe." The following chapters review the approach I take for my patients and their family members.

OVERVIEW OF TREATMENT
(SECTION 2, CHAPTERS 3–20)

"Things should be made as simple as possible, but not simpler."
—ALBERT EINSTEIN

It is likely that many of the interventions that are detailed in this book have not been mentioned during doctor's office visits. Why is this? Since the very beginning of my medical training, I always held in the back of my mind a lingering question, "What can I learn and what can I do to better the lives of patients with Alzheimer's disease?"

I gathered the perspectives of a variety of physicians, patients, caregivers, nurses, psychologists, and other allied healthcare professionals. I studied the scientific literature, read the journal articles, and attended neurologic research conferences and lectures throughout the United States and other parts of the world.

After completing my medical training, I decided to sub-specialize my clinical practice and focus 100% on Alzheimer's disease. Over these last fifteen years in medicine, I have put together a summation of what I have learned and what I have observed from treating patients and discussing the day-to-day realities of Alzheimer's disease with caregivers.

There are several ways to look at my overall philosophy of treating Alzheimer's disease. As a result of my personal experience and family history of AD, I try to treat my patients exactly the same way I would treat my own family members. I make my decisions by considering the risk-benefit ratio of any intervention. If the risk is low and potential for benefit is moderate or high, I suggest it. If a patient or caregiver is asking me to do "anything and everything, as long as it is generally safe," I listen to them. I give my best medical opinion to equip them with the tools they need to combat the disease. Several of the national and international AD experts that I have spoken with do not agree with every aspect of the approach I take. Several of these experts take the "societal perspective," as opposed to the "individual perspective" of AD patient care which I ascribe to.

For example, one of the recommendations that I make as an adjunct in my multimodal intervention plan for AD is suggesting specific dietary changes (e.g., low-carbohydrate, low saturated fat, high antioxidant), including eating fish high in omega-3 fatty acids. More specifically, the types of omega-3 fatty acids I teach my patients about are docosahexaenoic acid (DHA), along with lesser amounts of eicosapentaenoic acid (EPA). There are several studies that show the potential benefit of these omega-3s (via diet and/or supplements) in AD. However, eating fish high in DHA and EPA, and taking DHA/EPA supplements, have not been approved by the U.S. Food and Drug Administration (FDA) for AD treatment.

After reading the scientific studies and based on the evidence for effectiveness coupled with the relative safety, I began recommending that my patients make specific dietary changes (that include eating fish high in DHA and EPA), and consider complementing their diet with a nutritional supplement (in a capsule or liquid form). After a few years, I became convinced that this approach was well tolerated, reasonably priced, and seemed to be helpful as an adjunct in several patients, especially those in the earliest stages of Alzheimer's disease.

Again, if a patient or caregiver tells me, "I want to do anything and everything possible to fight this disease, as long as what you tell me to do is relatively safe," specific dietary changes (detailed in later chapters) and fish oil supplements (DHA more than EPA) will be part of my intervention. For these patients, based on my clinical experience, the scientific data, and relative safety, I suggest changes like increasing dietary omega-3s from fish, combined with one of three specific types of supplements (capsules or liquid) with which I have the most experience.

Granted, at the time of publication of this book, there have not been enough well-designed scientific studies (prospective, randomized, double-blinded, placebo-controlled trials) that allow clinicians to say with 100% certainty which AD patients, if any, will surely respond to DHA. The most recent study was published in the *Journal of the American Medical Association* in November 2010. This study used fish oil derived from algae and found that 2 grams of DHA alone did not help every patient (when looked at as a group), but it *did* help a subset of patients with a specific genetic makeup (APOE4 negative, more on this later). Up to 45% of AD patients are APOE4 negative, and as such, even if I have not performed genetic testing, I recommend this intervention (especially in the earliest stages of the disease) in my practice.

Until more studies are performed, the FDA will not allow physicians to prescribe DHA for AD. There are also no studies that compare the cost of taking these supplements with the amount of cost-savings to the patient and/or healthcare system, by improving quality of care. There is a wide variety of pricing on fish oil (with the most optimal brands of high-strength DHA capsules costing approximately twenty to twenty-five dollars per month, and liquid DHA approximately thirty per month). As such, many of my esteemed colleagues, and perhaps some of the doctors who are caring for you or your loved one, do not recommend eating fish or taking DHA/EPA supplements (nor do they usually recommend against it).

Another reason that many have not heard about some of these interventions is that the treating doctor likely doesn't have sufficient time to explain in detail all of the potential treatment options, and educate patients and caregivers about the disease. In an academic setting, I am very, very fortunate as I have an hour (or more) for every patient I see. At least half of this visit is spent solely on discussing treatment options, weighing the risks and benefits, and educating patients and caregivers about how to most optimally care for their disease.

Based on my clinical experience, it seems that by utilizing this multimodal Alzheimer's care plan, my patients tend to do better (especially in the first few years after diagnosis), than the standard population of patients that has been reported on. Why is this? While I do not have scientific data proving my multidisciplinary approach is better than "standard" care, I can honestly say that:

1. This is the exact care plan that I would offer to my own family members.

2. I have recommended this plan to countless patients over the years with a great deal of success and patient/caregiver satisfaction.

3. All recommendations are grounded in a fair degree of scientific evidence and favorable risk-benefit ratio.

4. These suggestions follow my patient and caregiver requests to offer "anything and everything possible" that has the potential for benefit against AD.

It is my firm belief that the options we cover in Chapters 3–20 will give the greatest potential for success in the fight against AD. While we have not yet found the "magic bullet" or "magic pill" to cure AD, I am sure that in the future the fight against Alzheimer's disease is a battle we can win.

Author Disclosure: Dr. Isaacson has served as a paid scientific advisor/consultant for companies that sell the FDA-approved cholinesterase inhibitor medications, the FDA-regulated medical food, and the website www.therapyformemory.com.

OVERVIEW OF PREVENTION
(SECTION 3, CHAPTERS 21–30)

"Firm conclusions cannot be drawn about the association of any modifiable risk factor with cognitive decline or AD."

—NIH STATE-OF-THE-SCIENCE CONFERENCE, APRIL 2010

It seems quite contradictory that you are about to read a section of a book entitled "Preventing Alzheimer's" after reading the quote above. The National Institutes of Health (NIH) came to the conclusion that as of April 2010, no firm recommendations can be made that will surely decrease the likelihood of developing AD.

It goes without saying that I disagree with the quote above. Dr. Carl Sagan, the great American scientist, writer, and astronomer summarized my vantage point in the following quote: "The absence of evidence does not imply evidence of absence." The NIH and FDA have been charged with the more than insurmountable task of not only trying to help us, but also protecting us from harm. As such, without definitive evidence, these national agencies are not able to come to conclusions about preventing cognitive decline or AD. As discussed earlier, if an individual asks me if there is anything he or she can do to lower their risk of developing AD, or at least anything that can be done to potentially delay the onset of symptoms, I will respond with the exact recommendations detailed in this section. This point is discussed again in greater detail in Chapter 1.

While I can by no means be sure that any one of these recommendations will 100% stop or delay the onset of AD, based on the favorable risk-benefit ratio and on the available scientific evidence, these are the exact same recommendations that I have made to my own patients and relatives of patients suffering from AD. I would also make these same suggestions to my own family members and friends.

Will there ever be a drug to prevent AD? Not in the near future, by no means in the next five years, and likely much longer (if ever). The legal definition of a drug, in summary, is an article intended for use in the diagnosis, cure, mitigation, treatment, or prevention of disease. The usual drug-approval process that needs to occur takes many, many years (from drug development to final FDA approval). This is due to the fact that there needs to be substantial evidence that the drug will have the effect it purports. In general, a drug designed to prevent a condition like AD needs to be extremely safe, because some people will be exposed only to the risk of the drug (since they may never actually get the disease).

Some in the healthcare field feel that finding a drug that stops cognitive aging brings about several social and ethical issues. They feel so strongly about this that it may even prevent the approval of a drug in the future to avoid people from becoming cognitively "supernormal."

I was recently at a lecture by one of the "higher ups" at the FDA. While I have the utmost professional respect for this individual, it is this individual's feeling that the long-term risks of slowing down or preventing cognitive decline is not worth the potential for side effects. Again, I respectfully disagree with this. In both the areas of Alzheimer's disease and cognitive aging in general, I strongly support doing anything and everything with a favorable risk-benefit ratio.

My prevention plan is philosophically quite similar to my AD treatment plan that is detailed in Section 2. My prevention plan focuses more on lifestyle modifications that are best begun sooner, rather than later, and are likely advisable beginning at least by the fourth decade of life. My plan also relies on dietary changes (as detailed in Chapter 28), eating fish high in the omega-3 fatty acid DHA, and taking DHA supplements (via capsule or liquid). As discussed in the treatment introduction earlier, there is some evidence that shows that DHA supplementation may slow cognitive decline in mild Alzheimer's patients who have a specific genetic makeup. When it comes to prevention, there is epidemiological data that suggests that specific dietary changes (e.g., Mediterranean-style; fish high in DHA/EPA; low-carbohydrate) may be helpful, and some recent data (published in November 2010 in *Alzheimer's and Dementia*, the journal of the Alzheimer's Association) that showed adults over the age of 55 with age-related cognitive decline demonstrated improvements in memory skills after taking 900 mg algae-based DHA supplements each day. While there is much research that needs to be done to replicate these findings and clarify which types of diets and fish oils work best, scientific evidence has led me to recommend these changes to patients at risk for AD.

While there are several key considerations for prevention, I give much attention to diet and social/physical activity. We will review studies showing that these interventions may be protective to the brain and delay the development of AD. As an example, diet and behavioral enrichment have been studied in both humans and animals. In December 2010, Krikorian and colleagues published a study comparing a high-carbohydrate diet vs. a very low-carbohydrate diet in patients with mild cognitive impairment (*Neurobiology of Aging*). This was a randomized trial of 23 patients over 6 weeks. This study showed significant benefits in the low-carbo-hydrate group in verbal memory, in addition to weight loss, decreased waist circumference, decreased fasting blood sugar, and decreased fasting insulin. While further studies are warranted to determine preventative potential and to investigate the bio-logical reasons why these dietary changes may work, this exciting evidence lends support to the dietary suggestions I make to my patients at risk. In animals, dogs (beagles) can be used as a "model" to study AD. As dogs get older, they have increasing susceptibility to "doggie Alzheimer's" or canine cognitive dysfunction syndrome. These dogs develop symptoms similar to humans (although I would not expect them to be losing their keys or misplacing their cell phones!), and also have pathology in the brain that is similar, but not identical (beta-amyloid protein deposition) to humans.

One study conducted over three years by Dr. Carl Cotman and colleagues at the University of California at Irvine looked at whether nutrition and diet interventions could possibly reduce aging in the brain and protect cognition in dogs. The study investigators wanted to determine whether dietary antioxidants would reduce oxidative damage in the brain cells. The antioxidant diet had several of the antioxidants that will be recommended later (e.g., spinach) as well as other supplements that were chosen to help protect the mitochondria (which is the part of the cell responsible for energy metabolism and is affected in AD). In addition to the dietary changes, exercise was included (three times per week walking and running) and increased socialization (dogs could exercise and play together).

By the second year of their study, it was apparent that the diet and behavior intervention was working. By year three, the intervention group (combination of diet and exercise/socialization) maintained thinking skills but the other group's thinking skills declined (nearly 80% of the dogs could no longer maintain their prior cognitive function). In fact, the animals in the intervention group regained the capacity to perform a task that they could only do when they were younger. On a neurobiological level, the intervention group had less oxidative damage in the brain cells and had an increase in efficiency of the respiratory chain. Antioxidant defense enzymes were also increased, which correlated with cognitive test results. Increases in an important protein called brain-derived neurotrophic factor (BDNF) was also most pronounced in the treatment group and approached the levels found in younger animals. BDNF is extremely important as this protein helps support survival of brain cells and encourages the growth of new brain cells and brain connections. BDNF is active in the area of the brain that is most responsible for memory, called the hippocampus. These studies were published in the *Journal of Neuroscience*, and *Neurobiology of Aging*, by Dr. Cotman and colleagues.

The take-home message of this research is that the combination of exercise and behavioral enrichment synergizes with diet to optimize brain health and cognitive performance. Integrating socialization elements into exercise may turn out to be a key factor, although this aspect needs further study. Translating these findings to humans is necessary and will take several years, but why wait? We will cover several lifestyle changes that can be made (with the approval of and review by the treating physician) that may reduce the likelihood of developing Alzheimer's or delay the onset of symptoms of cognitive decline.

Changing behaviors, especially lifelong behaviors, can be quite difficult, but not impossible. I literally have to beg and plead with some of my patients to exercise and eat better. I care for a 68-year-old recently retired physician, who came to see me at the urging of his wife due to "cognitive changes." She was worried since his father had a diagnosis of Alzheimer's, and she wanted to make sure he was not developing the earliest signs of AD. After a thorough workup and evaluation, everything was normal, although his wife asked whether there was anything he could do to possibly reduce the risk of getting AD in the future. I wrote him a prescription and told him to stick it on his refrigerator. What did I write on it? Exercise! Three to four times a week, for 30–45 minutes each session, Refills: 100.

A few weeks later, his wife called me to let me know that he refused to start exercising. I spoke with him on the telephone and did my best to encourage him to increase his activity level, including getting a personal trainer once or twice a week to help get the process going.

A few weeks later, I called his wife to see how things were going. Not surprisingly, he still would not follow my instructions. His next follow-up visit was scheduled for a few months later, and this time I asked the patient to bring both his wife and his daughter (also a physician) to the next visit. The patient agreed. When the day of his visit arrived, I was confident that with the help of the family, and a personal trainer, we could finally start making some progress.

The visit came. His wife and daughter did not show up to the appointment. The patient was still refusing to do anything I had asked him to do. So I fired the patient from my practice.

It is unfortunate that the situation had to come to this, but in retrospect, I am glad it happened. This event was the motivating spark to get things back on track. A few hours later, I received an apologetic phone call from his wife. The next day, I received a similar phone call from his daughter. At the next visit, his wife and all three children came (including two flying in from out of state). I spent over an hour and a half with the entire immediate family reviewing my prevention plan. Over the next several months, and to the shock of the family, the patient not only started to exercise, but he also started eating better (as per my recommendations). Not only did the patient feel better, but his wife felt that his thinking skills had also started to go back to normal! Regular exercise, improved diet, and structured activities led to more energy, a brighter mood, and sharper memory. In fact, both the patient and entire family adopted my recommendations. Three years later, the patient is still "normal," and family members are now invested in the care of their dad.

For those readers who have difficulty sticking to some of these recommendations or have trouble motivating their loved ones to stick to aspects of "the plan," I suggest a number of helpful tips. First, get the help of a qualified healthcare professional and schedule regular follow-up visits. Some may benefit from the assistance of a personal trainer, counselor, dietician, or life coach. Getting family members involved and using each other for motivation is one of the best ways—healthy family/group dinners, exercise sessions, and social activities will help to keep the group engaged. Remember the saying, "Rome wasn't built in a day." Try to choose one or two aspects to focus on, start slowly, and realize that efforts now will absolutely be worth the reward later. There is no better investment than in the health of oneself or in the ones you care about!

1. What are the best strategies for treating and preventing Alzheimer's Disease?

I take a fairly comprehensive approach in treating and preventing Alzheimer's disease that is different from many other physicians. I tell my patients that the recommendations I give to them would be the same exact recommendations I would give to my own family member, and I really mean that. There is no one magic pill or cure for Alzheimer's. I feel that from my clinical experience and based on the available scientific evidence, there are several pharmacologic (e.g., drugs, supplements) and non-pharmacologic interventions (e.g., diet, exercise) that are beneficial. Safety is of paramount importance; most of the treatment and prevention strategies that I recommend are generally safe, and each has some degree of evidence for effectiveness. Many physicians feel that they need extensive research to prove effectiveness of an intervention before recommending it. The "gold standard" for this research is usually conducted in a type of trial known as a randomized, double-blind, placebo-controlled trial. I agree with this statement. However, there is one important caveat: many of these trials have not been done yet, are difficult or expensive to conduct, and may not be conducted for several years, if ever. I try to balance the scientific evidence (called "evidence-based medicine") with observations from my clinical practice over the years, something I refer to as "experience-based" practice. For more information on this philosophy, please read the introduction to Section 1.

Dr. Louis Caplan, professor of neurology at Harvard Medical School, was one of the most influential figures in my development as a physician. I spent time with Dr. Caplan first as a medical student in 1999, again as a neurology resident (2002–2005), and most recently when I was invited back to speak at the Harvard Medical School "Grand Rounds" in Neurology at the Harvard Medical Institute in June 2011. I am privileged to have spent this time professionally with Dr. Caplan, but the most fun I have had in his company has actually been outside of the hospital setting. First, when we won a contest to play a game of softball at Fenway Park in 2004 (not easy for a devoted N.Y. Yankees fan!) and later at a New England Patriots vs. Miami Dolphins football game in 2009. (I'm actually a big N.Y. Jets fan so I stayed neutral as to the outcome of the game.) To say that Dr. Caplan has taught me a lot about the art and science of medicine over these ten years is an understatement.

Dr. Caplan wrote an article in *Reviews in Neurological Diseases* (2007) entitled "How well does 'evidence-based' medicine help neurologists care for individual patients?" In this article, he states that those who advocate for evidence-based medicine have established a prerequisite for what they con- sider trustworthy evidence: the randomized, dou- ble-blind, controlled trial and/or systematic reviews (or meta-analysis) of several randomized, controlled research trials. However, Dr. Caplan states (and I wholeheartedly agree) that evidence from large therapeutic trials cannot always be applied to the care of individual patients. These studies yield information only on the likely benefit of a particular treatment strategy (e.g., an experi- mental drug) among a large group of often hetero- geneous patients with a given disease or condition. Some trials may turn out positive, but these results may be of little or no practical benefit for most patients with the specific condition studied. Other studies may show that a certain treatment is bene- ficial, although it may have other risks and cause harm in other patients with the same condition.

Again, I feel that "sticking to the books" and strictly following only what has been scientifically proven may be doing patients a disservice. I agree with Dr. Caplan that physicians "should spend more time finding out what is wrong with each patient and getting to know his or her circumstances, family situations, psychosocial and economic stresses, thoughts, fears, biases, and wishes." Considering these aspects, only then can a physician use his or her best scientific judgment, combined with the art of medicine, to make the soundest recommendations to those that they treat. It is with this philosophy, balancing the risks and benefits to each individual patient, upon which I base my treatment and prevention considerations.

The other important aspect about my comprehensive approach to Alzheimer's is the biological principle of synergy. I am a firm believer in this concept; there is a synergistic effect of using a combination of interventions for both treatment and prevention of AD. This concept is apparent across a variety of human conditions. For example, drinking alcohol slows your reflexes and impairs thinking skills. As such, individuals should not drink alcohol and operate heavy machinery or drive a car. However, if an individual is sleep deprived, talking on their cell phone, reading a text message, and drinking alcohol before driving, the synergistic effects of all of these negative aspects will significantly increase the likelihood of a car accident. The interventions detailed in Sections 2 and 3 emphasize the potential for positive synergy of combining treatment and prevention strategies. As an example, Chapter 5 focuses on ways to increase the effectiveness of AD drugs by adding a commonly available vitamin (folic acid).

There is both theoretical and scientific evidence that suggests following such a comprehensive plan could have much larger effects than any one component can provide alone. This aspect is another fundamental problem of clinical trials; such studies (randomized trials) generally try to find benefits of an intervention in isolation, rather than the combination of several at once. It is very difficult to scientifically study more than one intervention at a time as it becomes impossible to accurately determine which aspects were truly effective, which had no effect, and which potentially may have caused harm. The multimodal approach that I discuss builds upon many years of clinical experience with these methods.

Please note: Several of the strategies for treatment and prevention are essentially the same. For example, in my clinical practice I recommend a specific approach to nutrition that may have benefit across the spectrum of AD. While many readers will read this book from cover to cover, other readers may tend to focus on either the treatment or prevention content alone. As such, there is a good deal of information that is repeated almost verbatim in each section. This will ensure that readers will not miss any of the important information and will not have to go back and forth from section to section to read excerpts of content. If you happen to realize that the section you are reading is one of the parts generally repeated from an earlier section, feel free to skip ahead or re-read, whatever suits your learning style or interests.

2. What are some of the latest research advances in Alzheimer's disease?

We have continued to make great strides in our understanding of AD. In fact, the last year has brought about several advances. At the Alzheimer's Association International Conference (AAIC) 2011, researchers presented several new important findings. A new mathematical model of risk factors for AD suggested that reducing lifestyle-based behaviors (like many of those discussed in this book) by 25% could potentially prevent millions of AD cases throughout the world, and almost 500,000 in the United States (Barnes and colleagues). The risk factors that were considered included diabetes, mid-life high blood pressure, mid-life obesity, smoking, inadequate physical activity, low educational attainment, and depression. Modifying these risk factors may lower AD risk and, as we will cover later on, may also slow down the progression or severity of AD symptoms.

Another study tried to determine which factors were most significantly related to maintaining thinking skills as people age. These factors included low scores on measures of stress, anxiety, depression, and trauma (Steinberg and colleagues). We will talk more about the importance of this later in the book.

One of the actively studied therapies that is currently being researched is the drug bapineuzumab, which is a form of "passive immunotherapy" being tested for mild to moderate AD. While the effectiveness of this drug has not yet been determined, the most recent data has shown that bapineuzumab was generally well tolerated and side effects tended to be mild (Salloway and colleagues).

Another study presented at this conference helped to clarify the relationship between trauma to the brain and mild cognitive impairment (Yaffe and colleagues). Veterans who experienced traumatic brain injury showed more that two times the likelihood of developing dementia. Another study found that retired NFL football players were at an elevated risk of MCI when compared to non-athletes and were significantly younger than non-athletes with MCI (Randolph and colleagues). These findings underscore the importance of protecting the brain from trauma as much as possible, especially in those at risk of developing AD. Several months ago, I evaluated a 65-year-old former football player in my clinic. His wife, a nurse, had read the 2011 edition of this book and had implemented several of the suggestions under the supervision of his treating physician. His onset of symptoms was at the age of 60, and over the last five years, he has continued to slowly decline, albeit very slowly. He is one of the many patients in my practice with a history of repeated head trauma. It is encouraging that in 2011 (and more to come in future years), due to these study results, active changes have been made and continue to be made to protect those at risk (e.g., Ivy League colleges with football teams have minimized the maximum number of full contact practices each week).

One of readers of the 2011 edition of this book provided feedback and specifically asked if the next edition could include some of the latest research trends involving MCI. In addition to the new AD diagnostic criteria incorporating MCI mentioned earlier, another study presented at AAIC related to factors that predict conversion from MCI to AD. Patients with MCI may have problems with memory, communication skills, or other thinking skills that are noticeable, but do not affect activities of daily living. New research from six countries (United States, Australia, France, Germany, Sweden, and the United Kingdom) has shown that factors that may indicate the progression of MCI to AD include depression, anxiety, age, cardiovascular risk factors, and low educational levels. In such cases, a comprehensive diagnostic workup should be initiated, and interventions to treat the symptoms and slow the onset of AD should be considered. In my clinical experience, the earlier multimodal treatment begins, the better the patient outcomes.

~

After reading this book, if you would like to make suggestions on how to make future editions more helpful for you, please visit the website www.The ADplan.com/Survey and enter code FREE2013. Prior to release of the 2013 edition, we will randomly select 50 people who completed the survey, and send out a free copy of the book when it is released. (In addition, and as a special token of our thanks, we will enter you in a raffle for a $100 Amazon giftcard.) This book has been written for all of those on the "front lines" of AD: patients, caregivers, family members, and even healthcare providers. If there is something this book can do to better help you, we definitely want to know.

---

3. What types of treatments do you consider for your patients?

Multimodal therapy is essential for Alzheimer's disease. The two modalities that I focus on include pharmacologic and non-pharmacologic.

Pharmacologic Considerations

The pharmacologic agents that I consider fall into one of three main categories:

1. Drugs (or medications)

2. Supplements (or nutraceuticals)

3. Medical Foods

There are currently four commonly used FDA-approved drugs for the various stages of Alzheimer's disease. I also consider a number of supplements and most recently a medical food. While many of us are most familiar with FDA-approved drugs, it is important to review the similarities and differences between each of these treatments.

FDA-Approved Drugs

Prescription drugs are the most well-studied Alzheimer's treatments in terms of effectiveness and safety. The research into these drugs is reviewed by the Food and Drug Administration (FDA), which approves (or denies) the explicit indications that drugs may be used for. These Alzheimer's disease-specific claims must be supported by the most comprehensive and well-designed clinical and scientific studies. These studies are designed to highlight potential safety issues, while also being pre-approved by the FDA. FDA-approved drugs have an information sheet called the package insert (PI) that contains valuable information. Patients should read and follow the recommendations detailed in the PI and discuss any questions about drug administration directly with their treating physician.

A prescription drug can make claims of "curing, treating, preventing, or mitigating the effects of symptoms of a specific disease." In order to obtain a drug, patients must get a prescription from their physician and have it filled by a licensed pharmacist.

Supplements

Dietary supplements, also referred to as nutraceuticals, are products that do not require a prescription from a physician, and are intended to supplement the diet and maintain good health and regular function. Supplements are usually available from a variety of sources, including supermarkets, health food stores, drugstores, and on the Internet. A supplement can contain any one or the combination of the following ingredients: vitamins, minerals, herbs or other botanicals, amino acids, dietary substances used to supplement the diet by increasing the total dietary intake (e.g., enzymes from tissues or organs), or a concentrate, metabolite, constituent, or extract.

When looking at the label of any supplement that makes a claim of an effect on structure or function of the body, expect to find the following: "This statement has not been evaluated by the FDA. This product is not intended to diagnose, treat, cure, or prevent any disease." For additional information, read about the term "dietary supplement" as defined by the Dietary Supplement Health and Education Act (DSHEA) of 1994.

Medical Food

As defined by the Orphan Drug Act (1988 Amendment), a medical food is "a food which is formulated to be consumed or administered orally under the supervision of a physician, and which is intended for specific dietary management of a disease or condition for which distinctive nutritional requirements, based on recognized scientific principles, are established by medical evaluation."

These therapeutic agents are a heterogeneous group of formulations that comprise a relatively new category of medical protocols defined by Congress and are subject to regulation by the FDA.

Medical foods achieve the "Generally Recognized As Safe" (GRAS) designation, the highest FDA standard of safety given to foods, which all components of the formulation must satisfy. Additionally, and unlike over-the-counter dietary supplements, they require the supervision and prescription of a physician.

Medical foods and dietary supplements are discrete classifications and are not interchangeable. Medical foods must be shown, by medical evaluation, to meet the distinctive nutritional needs of a specific, diseased patient population being targeted prior to marketing. In contrast, dietary supplements are intended for normal, healthy adults and require no pre-market efficacy tests. In addition, medical foods require *physician supervision* and a *prescription.*

To summarize, medical foods are medical products for a specific nutritional purpose, as opposed to dietary supplements, which are a consumer product to supplement the diet and maintain good health and regular function.

Non-Pharmacologic Considerations

I also consider several non-pharmacologic approaches. Some examples include physical and mental exercise, music therapy, and diet modification. These are covered in greater detail later in the book.

Also, while unproven, there are several interventions that may help in the fight against AD by protecting brain cells. Certain dietary or lifestyle changes can decrease damage in the cells known as "oxidative stress." Reducing this type of stress in the brain may be protective against AD. For example, substances with "antioxidant" properties need to be further studied in large, randomized, double-blind, placebo-controlled trials. While there is a lack of clear evidence in humans, there is evidence in animals that these agents have potential benefits and, for the most part, are also quite safe.

4. What are the drug treatment considerations for Alzheimer's?

The first class of FDA-approved medications aim to increase the chemical in the brain that is primarily responsible for memory. The name of this chemical is called acetylcholine, and these medications help stop its breakdown in the brain. As such, they are called cholinesterase inhibitors, or in simpler terms, "memory chemical breakdown" inhibitors. There are three commonly used drugs in this category and each has specific characteristics that physicians consider when prescribing for individual patients.

It is important to note that these medications work differently in different patients, and my definition of "success" does not always have to mean a "big" improvement. I am happy when patients improve, but I am also satisfied when patients begin to stabilize while on these treatments. From my clinical experience, roughly 30–40% of patients on these medications improve, 30% stay at the same baseline, and 30% continue to decline. Since it is impossible to tell which patient may respond, I am an advocate for treatment (as there is an acceptable risk-benefit ratio that needs to be discussed in detail with the patient's physician).

All medications have some degree of risk, and patients and caregivers should understand these side effects in detail. In an ideal world, the physician would educate patients and caregivers at length about not only how the medications work, but also how to minimize side effects by using these agents most effectively. In general, the "start low and go slow" approach is usually best—remember, this disease develops over many years and continues for a long time after diagnosis, so there is no rush in starting medications too quickly. Starting at high doses may increase the likelihood of side effects. If a patient does experience a side effect to any medication, the physician should be contacted as the administration schedule or dose may need to be changed, the medication may need to be stopped entirely, or in some cases medical attention must be sought immediately. As with any medical emergency, if there is a question about the seriousness of any side effect or any medical illness in general, the patient or caregiver should call 911 immediately, and the patient should be evaluated in the nearest emergency room. Importantly, and as mentioned in Chapter 3, it is essential to read and follow guidelines written in the drug PI and discuss drug administration instructions and safety with the treating physician.

In 2007, the newest formulation of medications in this class was released called the rivastigmine (Exelon) patch. In my patients, I recommend starting the Exelon patch at 4.6 mg each day for four weeks, which is the smallest dose. If this is tolerated, the dosage can then be increased to a 9.5 mg patch. Caution should be used in patients who weigh less than 110 pounds (50 kg) as using the higher dose of the patch in these patients may increase side effects. There is also the likelihood that a higher dose of the patch may be released. The 13.3 mg patch has been tested in ongoing clinical trials (including the OPTIMA trial), and the FDA will be reviewing the research and will make a determination based on the results.

The patch should be placed on the upper back (see the picture in the PI, which identifies appropriate locations to place the patch) to clean, dry, hairless, and intact skin. The application site should be rotated each day to reduce the possibility of skin irritation, and the same exact spot should not be used within 14 days. It is also essential to be sure that after 24 hours, the old patch is removed from the skin, as having multiple patches on at the same time can cause significant side effects (e.g., slow heart rate, loss of consciousness, or death).

Using this medication in a patch form may reduce side effects since it bypasses the gastrointestinal system, or stomach. In the past, Exelon needed to be given with a full meal in order to reduce the likelihood of side effects like diarrhea, nausea, and vomiting. Patients may still have side effects from the patch and should still be encouraged to eat a balanced diet (more on this in later chapters) as instructed by their primary care physician.

The oral medication in this class that is most commonly used is called donepezil (Aricept). Aricept is usually started at 5 mg each day with food, and in my patients, I always suggest taking it with either breakfast or lunch, whichever meal is bigger. After 4 weeks, Aricept should be increased to 10 mg each day if tolerated. Some physicians do not suggest taking the medication at night as there is a slight increased risk of having either vivid dreams or nightmares. That being said, several patients do take Aricept at night and have neither of these side effects. In my clinical practice, if a patient is taking the medication at night and tolerating it without side effects, I do not suggest changing the time of dose. If side effects do occur, it is advisable to discuss the time of administration with the treating physician.

Aricept is the only medication in this class available in an oral disintegrating tablet (ODT) for patients who have difficulty swallowing. When patients do have swallowing difficulty, also known as "dysphagia," I will preferentially consider the Exelon patch or Aricept ODT in my practice.

In August 2010, a higher strength of Aricept was released. Aricept 23 mg was approved for use in severe dementia (see the PI for more information). In my clinical practice, I will consider increasing the dose to 23 mg in patients who have been tolerating the 10 mg tablet for at least 3 months. If this medication is increased from 10 mg to 23 mg, it is imperative to stress that the patient takes it with a full meal or as directed by the prescribing physician. In December 2010, the oral form of donepezil was released as a generic medication.

Another oral medication option is galantamine (Razadyne ER). This is also available as a generic and, like donepezil, is a valuable option for patients who have difficulty affording their medications. Razadyne ER should be started once a day at 8 mg and taken with a full meal in the morning or at lunch. Razadyne ER can be increased monthly to 16 mg per day, and if tolerated, 24 mg per day as the maximum dose (four weeks after increasing to 16 mg).

As the disease progresses, I often consider adding memantine (Namenda) in combination with a cholinesterase inhibitor in my clinical practice. Namenda is approved by the FDA for moderate to severe AD since it has been shown in clinical trials to be efficacious in this patient population. Namenda works via a different neurochemical pathway when compared to the cholinesterase inhibitors (NMDA-antagonist). This medication should also be started slowly, to the maximum recommended dose of 10 mg twice a day. In my patients, I have had the most success with starting Namenda once a day at 5 mg with or without food. At 1-week intervals, the dose should be increased first to 5 mg twice a day, then to 5 mg for the first dose of the day and 10 mg for the second dose of the day. Finally, if tolerated, it should be increased to 10 mg two times a day. As with the other medications above, doses may be skipped or the drug dosage reduced if a side effect occurs, and any side effect must be discussed with the prescribing physician. After lowering the dose, the treating physician may suggest a higher dose to be tried again at a later date.

Some physicians have used Namenda "off-label," meaning not only in patients with moderate to severe disease, and not in line with instructions detailed in the PI. Some recent scientific data suggests that Namenda may have some benefit in patients with mild disease, but only when used in combination with a cholinesterase inhibitor. The decision to begin Namenda earlier than the FDA-approved indication should be left up to the patient's treating physician. In my clinical practice, I have used Namenda in earlier stage disease in combination with a cholinesterase inhibitor with success. However, this indication is not FDA approved, and this decision must be made by the treating physician. Namenda XR was approved by the FDA as a once-a-day pill (28 mg), and there is the possibility that it will be available by prescription in 2012.

All of the FDA-approved drugs have associated costs. The exact amount may depend on type of insurance coverage (if any), co-pay amount, pharmacy pricing/location, availability as a generic medication, and a variety of other factors. Without insurance coverage, these medications may cost (on average) of $125 to $200 per month for the brand-name medications. Generics drugs (as of 2011, galantamine and donepezil) may be significantly cheaper (less than half). Average insurance co-payments for brand-name drugs are usually higher ($30–$55 per month) as compared with generic drugs ($10–$20 per month). There is often a price difference between pharmacies, even those located in the same city, or even on the same street! It is sensible to call several pharmacies, discuss with other caregivers, a social worker, or staff at the treating physician's office.

The monetary costs of drugs need to be balanced with potential for benefit. For example, there are studies on combination therapy with cholinesterase inhibitors and Namenda that show caregivers may in fact need to spend less time each month with patient supervision and care.

Less time caregiving means less stress and less associated costs, which help to balance the cost of the drugs at the pharmacy. Additional studies have shown that as the disease progresses, combination drug therapy may even delay nursing-home placement for over a year. That cost savings alone can balance out the drug costs of many years of treatment.

5. What can I do to increase the effectiveness of Alzheimer's medications?

In my clinical practice, I almost always start the vitamin folic acid 1 mg with a cholinesterase inhibitor (Aricept [donepezil], Exelon [rivastigmine], and Razadyne [galantamine]). There was one small research study that showed increased clinical benefit of the cholinesterase medications when folic acid was used in combination (*International Journal of Geriatric Psychiatry*, 2008). This was one small study that will need to be repeated, but since folic acid is relatively safe, I do tend to recommend it. Like all interventions, adding this vitamin to a patient's treatment plan needs to be discussed and approved by the treating physician.

Another way to ensure optimal effectiveness of drugs is to take them as directed and try to not miss any doses. Missing doses for several days or several weeks can have a significant negative effect. In fact, in several of my patients, restarting the medications after not taking them for many weeks did not bring the patient back to the same level as before they stopped taking them. I thus advocate for the caregiver and patient to work together to ensure that doses are not missed. When necessary, a home healthcare nurse may be suggested by the treating physician. The nurse will make periodic home visits to help with medication administration and record keeping.

6. What can I do to decrease the side effects of Alzheimer's medications?

For each of the cholinesterase inhibitor medications (Aricept [donepezil], Exelon [rivastigmine], and Razadyne [galantamine]), if side effects occur when the dose has been increased, the treating physician may suggest to decrease the dose back to a lower strength.

Based on the clinical trial data, I do not feel that the 4.6 mg dose of the Exelon patch is sufficient if a patient is unable to tolerate the 9.5 mg patch. In this case, the treating physician may switch to an alternative medication. However, the 4.6 mg dose of the Exelon patch may be sufficient for patients who weigh less than 110 pounds, and this decision should be discussed with the treating physician. I am occasionally asked if it is advisable to cut the 9.5 mg patch in half to approximate the 4.6 mg does. I advise against cutting the patch as it has not been studied in clinical trials.

With Aricept, if side effects are experienced, it is important to ensure that the dose was taken correctly (with a big meal, either breakfast or lunch). It is preferable to have some fat in the meal as this may increase tolerability. If side effects occur after increasing to the 10 mg dose, reducing the dose back down to 5 mg may be suggested for a few days, and a re-trial of 7.5 mg (one and a half tablets of 5 mg) may be considered in the future instead of increasing to 10 mg. If the treating physician suggests a subsequent increase to 23 mg, it may be best tolerated after at least three months on the 10 mg dose and after a big meal.

With Razadyne ER, if a side effect is experienced with the 24 mg per day dose, it is again important to ensure that the dose was taken correctly (with a big meal, either breakfast or lunch). The minimum therapeutic dose is 16 mg per day, and as such, if a patient can only tolerate the 8 mg per day dose, the treating physician may decide to switch to different medication in this category.

In general, if a side effect occurs with any of these treatments, doses may be skipped or drug dosage reduced until the negative effects disappear, and a higher dosage may be tried again at a later date. Positive effects on memory, thinking skills, functioning of everyday activities, and behavior may be countered by adverse side effects such as nausea, vomiting, and diarrhea, which also become more likely with dosage increases. It is important to find a favorable balance between side effects and the overall effectiveness of the medication.

If patients do not tolerate one cholinesterase inhibitor, they may tolerate another, so the treating physician may consider a switch. Also, if one cholinesterase inhibitor is not effective or the patient continues to decline, the physician may consider switching to an alternative medication.

7. What supplements do you consider and what is the evidence that they work?

There are two specific supplements that I routinely recommend. These include fish oil (omega-3 fatty acids, specifically DHA and EPA) and curcumin (turmeric root).

Fish oil has been studied in a variety of scientific trials, and there is evidence for its usefulness in Alzheimer's. There is some evidence that using specific types of fish oil may not only have a treatment benefit in the most mildly affected patients (Freund-Levi, 2006), but also may possibly slow down the progression of the disease.

I want to clarify a few aspects about fish oil—there are different types that are most commonly known about such as omega-3 fatty acids and omega-6 fatty acids. While there is still much research to be done in order to determine which types work best, in my clinical practice, I prefer to consider the omega-3s, mainly docosahexaenoic acid (DHA) and eicosapentaenoic acid (EPA).

In the supermarket, neighborhood drugstore, health food store, and on the Internet, there are many types of fish oil available for sale. It is important to note that all fish oil is not created equal. The most common type that is available will say "Fish Oil 1,000 mg" on the label. For Alzheimer's disease, it is essential to take the right type of capsules. One must look at the label and see the breakdown of how much DHA and EPA are in each capsule, and how many capsules are needed for each serving size. Oftentimes, one will need to take at least several capsules each day in order to get a suitable amount of these two omega-3 fatty acids.

In general, I recommend that patients with Alzheimer's (most especially early Alzheimer's) consider taking fish oil. When selecting from different varieties, I suggest those made up of more DHA than EPA, with at least 250 mg of DHA in each capsule (and a total of at least 1,000–1,500 mg daily of DHA specifically). Fish oil supplementation should be started only under the supervision of a physician, and patients should begin with one capsule each day with a big meal and with water or juice, then increase if tolerated to one capsule twice per day over a week or so. Just like the cholinesterase medications above, it is suggested to start low and increase slowly.

The most recent research has shown that it may be necessary for patients to take even higher amounts of DHA, such as 1,500–2,000 mg each day. I base this on one study mentioned above published in *Archives of Neurology* in 2006 (DHA 1,720 mg and EPA 600 mg each day) that showed benefits, and another more recent trial that was performed by the Alzheimer's Disease Cooperative Study (more on this later). In order to get this high amount of DHA, I tend to recommend a brand called Carlson Super DHA Gems, which have 500 mg of DHA per capsule; another brand is Life's DHA (made by Martek, and derived from algae—not fish), but any brand with a high DHA is suggested.

Like the FDA-approved drugs, the cost of these supplements will depend on a variety of factors. The price most significantly depends on the brand or strength of the fish oil and the location purchased. There is often a price difference between pharmacies in the same city, and on Internet websites. It is advisable to shop around and visit several pharmacies, health food stores, and websites, and discuss with other caregivers, a social worker, or staff at the treating physician's office. It is imperative to pay close attention to the exact brand name, strength of each capsule, and serving size. The average cost of Carlson Super DHA Gems ranges from $30–$35 for 180 capsules, or $20–$25 per month (1,500 mg total DHA per day, 500 mg capsules), and the average cost of Life's DHA by Martek ranges from $22–$30 for 90 capsules, or $50 per month (1,800 mg total DHA per day, 300 mg capsules).

The most recent study on fish oil was published in the *Journal of the American Medical Association* in November 2010. This study used fish oil derived from algae (made by Martek) and found that 2,000 mg of DHA alone did not help patients when looked at as a group, but *did* help a subset of patients with a specific genetic makeup (APOE4 negative, see Chapter 21 in Section 3 for more details about genetics and Alzheimer's disease).

Up to 45% of AD patients are APOE4 negative, and as such, even if I have not performed genetic testing, I recommend using any of the brands above.

Again, fish oil capsules usually have a varying amount (e.g., 1,000 mg) of *total* fish oil in each capsule, but each has a different amount of actual DHA and EPA. As an alternative to capsules, a liquid fish oil may be used. One brand to consider is called Nutri Supreme (available online at www.nutri-supreme.com or by calling 1-888-68-NUTRI), which is also Kosher. For example, the average cost for a 12-ounce bottle of "Omega-3 GOLD" liquid fish oil (also contains 1,000 I.U. of vitamin D3 per teaspoon) is $43, or roughly $35 per month via the manufacturer's website.

Fish oil is generally safe but must be used under the supervision of a physician as there could be interactions with other medications. Fish oil may affect bleeding and should be used with caution in patients on an anticoagulant (blood thinner) medication like Coumadin (which means that a doctor should follow blood work closely). Overall, fish oil is relatively safe and also may have a beneficial effect on cholesterol, so I utilize this intervention frequently in my practice. Depending on the brand

and type of fish oil that is taken, some patients may experience side effects, like a "fish taste" after taking them. To minimize this, I sometimes suggest taking capsules toward the beginning of a meal, or in the middle of a meal, and with plenty of water or other liquids.

The other supplement that I often suggest is curcumin, also called turmeric root, which is the active ingredient in curry. There is no clear standardized dosing, and it is not currently known what dose or type is most beneficial.

There are ongoing scientific trials studying this treatment. Since curcumin supplementation seems generally safe and there is some data to suggest its usefulness, I do recommend it in my clinical practice. Usually curcumin supplements can be purchased in a health food store. I advise patients to follow the administration guidelines on the bottle. However, since supplements are not regulated by the FDA and all brands are different in terms of dosage/strength, it is unclear which brand is best. In terms of safety, it is essential to discuss taking this supplement with the treating physician as there may be some potential for interactions with prescribed medications. The costs of curcumin vary widely depending on vendor, dosage, and strength, on average of $10 to $15 per month.

One strategy that I use to optimize the effectiveness of curcumin is to suggest that my patients take each pill with a meal containing some fat or with a dose of fish oil. For example, I evaluated a patient recently and modified their medication schedule to take two 500 mg DHA capsules and one tablet of curcumin with breakfast, and another two capsules of fish oil and one tablet of curcumin with dinner.

8. What medical food do you consider and what is the evidence that it works?

Within the last few years, the first medical food for Alzheimer's disease was released. This food is supplied as a powder that is mixed with a liquid and consumed after a big meal (breakfast or lunch) once each day.

The name of this product is Axona, which contains caprylic triglyceride, a medium-chain triglyceride that is broken down by the liver into ketone bodies. Ketone bodies can be used by the brain as an alternative fuel source to glucose, which is the brain's usual energy supply. It has been known for some time that the brains of patients with AD have a decreased ability to use glucose, and thus ketone bodies may improve cognitive function. Based on the initial study (Henderson, 2009), Axona has been shown to have a positive effect on cognitive function in a specific group of patients (depends on genetic factors). Even more recent evidence shows that roughly 13% of APOE4 negative patients may have a dramatic increase in cognitive functioning (also most likely attributable to genetic factors).

Axona is only available with a prescription and must be used under the supervision of a physician. Since this is a relatively new product, and since medical foods are not commonly used by many physicians, some patients may have difficulty finding a practitioner who is familiar with it. If a patient has difficulty finding a prescriber, there is a list of doctors that have experience with it on the Axona website.

When starting Axona, it is again important to start low and go slow. In my clinical practice, I suggest that my patients start with either a quarter or a half packet per day with food (preferably breakfast or lunch, whichever meal is bigger) for a week and then increase slowly over a week or two to one full packet per day. The powder packet should be mixed with 6–8 ounces of water, meal replacement drink (e.g., Boost/Ensure), or other liquid (like skim milk or juice) to ensure tolerability and must only be taken after a meal. When the drink is being prepared, it is suggested to first pour 6–8 ounces of liquid into a shaker cup (if a patient gets a sample from their physician, there is usually a shaker cup included), and then the powder should be added to the liquid. The combination should then be shaken/blended (rather than stirred) to ensure tolerability. It is important to drink the mixture slowly over 20–30 minutes, and the company provides information printed on the sample box that gives helpful hints on how to improve tolerability.

Many patients find it easier to purchase several shaker cups as this will reduce the need to wash them on a daily basis. Some shaker cups come with mixing spheres or "agitators" that help to mix the powder into a more palatable form (purchase these types if possible).

The Axona sample kits that may be available from physicians have miniature packets that contain one-quarter of the full packet amount that is usually dispensed when a patient fills the prescription. The sample kits allow patients to gradually increase the dose of Axona, thus decreasing the likelihood of side effects when first starting the product. If a sample kit is not available and you instead fill a prescription, physicians may suggest starting at a lower dose. Some physicians suggest a quarter of a packet per day for a few days, then a half packet per day for a few days, then three-quarters of a packet per day for a few days, then increasing to the full packet as tolerated. Other physicians may begin at a half a packet per day for a week, then increasing to the full packet. Regardless of how your physician starts Axona, it is imperative to drink the mixture slowly after a big meal (breakfast or lunch) as described above.

Patients who have a history of milk or soy allergies, diabetic ketoacidosis, poorly controlled diabetes, or a variety of other health conditions should not take Axona. This product is generally safe, but as with all therapies, must be used under the close supervision of a physician. As discussed earlier, Axona has been tested in a phase-2 randomized, double-blind, placebo-controlled trial and was shown to be effective for a subset of patients who were negative for the APOE4 gene (see Chapter 21 in Section 3 for more information about APOE4). While genetic testing is only rarely done by physicians, most prescribers try Axona without ordering genetic testing. If after three months the patient continues to decline, most physicians will stop recommending it. In my clinical practice, I do not yet perform genetic testing for a variety of reasons (which go beyond the scope of this chapter).

The manufacturer has ongoing clinical trials, which are necessary, and more information can also be found online at the FDA clinical trials website (www.clinicaltrials.gov). Additional information may also be found on the company website. Since Axona is classified as a medical food (and not an FDA-approved drug), some insurance companies may not cover it. In such cases, the manufacture offers a 20% discount coupon that may be available on the website (www.about-axona.com) or via the physician's office. The cost (after discount) varies from pharmacy to pharmacy, so it is a good idea to check several. For example, I have one patient who pays $72/month, and another who pays $91/month from a different pharmacy in the same city, so it is sensible to check around.

If the future clinical trials are positive, the FDA may review these data and approve Axona as a drug. This would open the door to wider insurance coverage for many individuals.

In my clinical practice, I tend to suggest that my patients engage in a cognitively stimulating activity roughly two hours after drinking Axona. By this time, the ketone bodies have traveled to the brain and may give the brain more "fuel" to participate in activities. For example, I have one caregiver who takes her husband to the movies, and another caregiver who listens to a music activity and educational program on CD with his wife two hours after administration (see the next chapter and the website resources section at the end of the book for more information). Social interaction with family or friends is also a great option.

9. What non-pharmacologic interventions may be helpful and are these strategies really among the most effective in AD treatment?

I absolutely cannot stress enough the importance of physical exercise, as well as mental exercise, including music therapy.

The benefits of physical exercise on patients with Alzheimer's disease have been suggested in a variety of studies. There is also some very interesting research in lab animals (mice) that supports this. In one study, mice with "Alzheimer's disease" were put in two separate environments. Half the mice were very active and undertook physical exercise on a regular basis. The other mice did not have much physical activity at all. When the researchers looked at the brains of the mice that exercised, the level of the "bad" Alzheimer's protein in the brain was cut in half! Studies in humans have also shown the cognitive benefits of exercise.

Considering this, and based on my clinical experience, I am a strong advocate for increasing physical activity as tolerated and as approved by the patient's primary care physician. Oftentimes, I suggest a personal trainer if motivation is a problem. I suggest exercise at least 3–4 times a week, for 45–60 minutes if tolerated. However, it is important to gradually increase time spent exercising. As an example, if a patient does not get any exercise at all, even starting with a 5-minute walk once or twice a day is better than nothing. Ten minutes is better than five, twenty is better than ten, and so on. Some studies suggest that aerobic exercise is important, and other studies suggest that adding muscle mass via weight training is also helpful. Further research is warranted.

We do not have enough scientific evidence to tell which is better or in what combination, so I usually recommend a mixture of both, increasing as tolerated to the time periods listed above. When patients have mobility issues due to arthritis or other problems, pool therapy in a supervised environment is an option to consider.

Periodic mental activities may also be helpful.

Some suggestions that I recommend to my patients include video games like Brain Age and Big Brain Academy (available on the videogame systems Nintendo DS or Nintendo Wii), puzzles, word games, reading books, crosswords, and other games requiring thought. Some studies suggest that the more one challenges the brain, the more one will be able to maintain its function. There are several resources that may be helpful, including brain teaser books. One good website for brain activities that tracks patient progress is www.lumosity.com. I tell my patients that using this website once per week is generally a good idea to exercise the mind and track their progress.

While I advocate for brain games intermittently throughout the week, I usually do not overstress brain activity. Some researchers believe that doing the same brain activity over and over again (like Sudoku) only helps improve the patient's ability at doing that particular brain activity and not in other cognitive areas. Other researchers feel that "overdoing it" with focused brain games like Sudoku, and other mentally stimulating activities (especially games that frustrate the patient), may actually have a detrimental effect. Much research needs to be done in order to clarify this. There has been some interesting research in the area of gist reasoning, as this type of cognitive activity may "spill over" and help to improve cognitive skills in other areas. This topic will be discussed in greater detail later in the book.

The aspect of brain exercise that I most strongly advocate for is learning something new. Taking classes (e.g., adult education) and learning a new language or a new skill may be especially important. Finding new hobbies and getting involved in group activities that incorporate socialization are also quite important.

Listening to music (especially classical) and music therapy programs have been shown to improve memory in patients with Alzheimer's disease. Many individuals do not have access to a board-certified music therapist for music therapy sessions. As such, I suggest to my patients the innovative Therapy for Memory program available online at a website that I have recently been involved with called www.TherapyForMemory.com. The new Therapy for Memory program has been developed by a team of healthcare providers (e.g., neurologist, psychologist, nurse) and is produced by professionally trained musicians. The program incorporates a variety of mind-stimulating activities that builds upon years of research showing that music can be used to stimulate brain function.

Listening to music while sleeping has also been shown to stimulate brain function (as memories are consolidated, or formed, during sleep) and calm the listener during waking hours. On the website listed above, there is music available that can be listened to while sleeping. In addition, other one-on-one and group music therapy sessions are available in several areas of the country. Attending a musical performance, theater, or the symphony on a regular basis may be helpful. Learning how to play an instrument or practicing an instrument that one has played in the past may also be beneficial.

In addition to listening to the Therapy for Memory Activity and Educational Program on CD, there are a variety of ways to incorporate the power of music into the management plan for memory impairment.

Some suggestions to be considered include:

1. Set aside time every day to listen to favorite songs from childhood, high school, college years, early adulthood, and beyond. Try to listen to more upbeat familiar music either in the morning or afternoon for about 1 hour per day, and more relaxing familiar songs in the evening before bed.

2. Songs that remind listeners of familiar events in the past may help to rekindle memories of past events. Look at old pictures from those events while listening to the music for a more powerful result.

3. Play "guess the name of the song" by playing the beginning of old familiar tunes on the CD or record player at home. Also consider buying a variety of games, or search online for free games (here is one example using television tunes: www.television tunes.com/game.php).

4. Go to the symphony or a concert. Several communities all throughout the country offer free events throughout the year, and especially in the

summertime. Use the Internet to search for free concerts in your area, or check out the events calendar at your favorite venues. Better yet, join the email mailing list for these concert venues online.

5. Make a list of favorite artists, songs, and albums. Then create a library of music organized by decade. Buy digital recordings when possible, as these will last forever. Visit local music stores and look through favorite genres or artists' albums. It may be beneficial to talk about these albums and reminisce about the songs and time period when it was released. Read the liner notes, as this will show where and when the album was created and may trigger past memories.

6. Upgrade the stereo and speaker system. Try to get "surround sound" to maximize listening experience.

There is extensive scientific evidence for music therapy in AD. For a detailed listing of this research, or to watch a live demonstration of the music activity and educational program on CD, visit www.TherapyForMemory.com.

Benefits of music therapy have been found for memory, as well as attention/focus, language/speaking skills, behavior (anxiety, agitation, and depression), caregiver burden, sleep, and chemical regulation in the brain. Examples of research findings include significant improvements in anxiety and depression (effect of music therapy was sustained for up to 8 weeks after discontinuation); weight of the physical/emotional burden experienced by caregiver fell significantly; music therapy significantly improved performance on both speech content and fluency of spontaneous speech; significant increase in positive social behaviors and a significant decrease in negative behaviors related to agitation when music is played; and patients with Alzheimer's disease demonstrated better recognition accuracy for sung lyrics than spoken lyrics.

10. Are diet and nutrition important in the treatment of AD?

Yes! Maintaining a healthy diet is extremely important. Patients should be encouraged to utilize the combination of a balanced diet and good overall physical health, as they work together to optimize health status in Alzheimer's disease. Before making a dietary change, it should be discussed with, and approved by, the patient's primary care physician or a dietician.

Let's review important aspects of nutrition that should not be overlooked for patients with AD. While perhaps more important for long-term prevention, I also feel that based on recent scientific evidence, these suggestions are a very important part of the comprehensive treatment program for AD. There is still much research that needs to be done in the area of dietary intervention for AD. Unfortunately, this research is difficult to perform due to the long length of the studies and the many variables that come into play when studying nutritional techniques. In my clinical practice, I advocate several dietary changes to my patients. I ask that my patients complete diet log sheets to track what they eat (available for download on the website www.TheADplan.com). While most patients are able to make some positive changes to their diet habits, roughly 40% of my patients are able to stick to one of the most important aspects: lowering dietary carbohydrates.

Before we review which specific types of food and beverage choices are best, it is important to at least obtain a basic understanding of the fundamentals of AD nutrition, as it will help patients and caregivers make the right food choices. In the back of the book in the Resources section, there are several examples of food choices to consider. This section lists choices that may be better for optimal brain health. There is also a section on food terminology, to help with understanding of dietary choices in life. These sections were added to this edition based on feedback from readers like you. In fact, we received so much positive feedback about the diet and nutrition sections in this book that we are now working a new book focusing solely on diet and nutrition for AD. You can visit www .TheADdiet.com for more information, or to complete a reader survey about this book, please visit www.TheADplan.com/Survey. Your input and time are both greatly appreciated!

Last year, I had the pleasure of dining with a gentleman who has a doctorate degree (Ph.D.) in nutritional science. He also has a strong family history of AD. I asked him the following question: What is the number one thing that you would suggest for a patient with Alzheimer's? His response was simple: a low-carbohydrate diet, avoiding simple sugars. Now let's discuss what he meant by simple sugars, and then review the reasons why such diet modification may be important.

There are three different types of "macro" nutrients, which most people are familiar with. These include proteins, fats, and carbohydrates. Some examples of protein sources that I recommend for my patients with AD include fish high in DHA (e.g., wild salmon, mackerel, lake trout, herring, sardines, albacore tuna), poultry (skinless chicken and turkey), and lean meats (beef) that are hormone free when possible, egg whites, and low-fat (or better yet, non-fat) dairy products. Mono-saturated fats (e.g., extra-virgin olive oil, peanuts, avocados) and polyunsaturated fats (e.g., nuts and seeds) in moderation are advisable. Avoiding trans fats and saturated fats is of very high importance. I also suggest minimizing "simple sugars." As an example, simple sugars include the type of sugar people put in their coffee (cane sugar), as well as more concentrated versions such as high fructose corn syrup and corn syrup in general.

There are two different types of sugars: "added sugars" and "naturally occurring" sugars. An added sugar is a sugar or syrup that is added to foods during processing or preparation. These do not include naturally occurring sugars such as fructose (in fruits) or lactose (in milk products). All sugars/carbohydrates, regardless if they are added or naturally occurring, can be characterized in terms of their glycemic index.

The term "glycemic index" is important to understand. Just like the different types of fish oil described earlier, all carbohydrates are not created equal. Glycemic index refers to a classification proposed to quantify the relative blood glucose response to carbohydrate-containing foods (cited from www.health.gov). In other words, for the carbohydrate that is eaten (e.g., cane sugar vs. pasta), the glycemic index tells us how much a hormone (or a "regulatory substance") called insulin is released by the body in response.

There are several theories as to why minimizing dietary intake of carbohydrates may be useful. One theory relates to the production of ketone bodies, which can be used as an alternative fuel source for the brain and may help reduce oxidative damage inside brain cells (in mitochondria). This is covered in greater detail in Chapter 8.

Another theory is based on the role of insulin, especially as it relates to consumption of high glycemic index carbohydrates. Insulin's effects on aging of the brain have been studied in detail. Regulating insulin "signaling" affects longevity in every known animal species and has a role in normal and pathological brain aging (Barbieri, 2003). Insulin receptors are densely packed in the hippocampus (the memory center in the brain), and it has a direct influence on the brain since it enters the brain by crossing into the blood brain barrier (Apelt, 2001). It also modulates neurotransmitters in the brain and is involved with memory.

Insulin resistance is a condition where insulin cannot carry out its usual activities. Insulin resistance is associated with a variety of medical conditions, including obesity, diabetes, high blood pressure, and high cholesterol. In addition, insulin and beta-amyloid are related. Studies have shown that insulin raises beta-amyloid (the pathologic protein found in the brain of patients with Alzheimer's disease) in older adults (over 70 years old) and also increases brain inflammation (Watson, 2003).

Now that you understand more about the importance of insulin, it becomes easier to understand why minimizing simple carbohydrates is a sensible idea. Simple carbohydrates are composed of a single sugar molecule or two joined sugar molecules, such as glucose, fructose, lactose, and sucrose. Simple carbohydrates include white and brown sugar, fruit sugar, corn syrup, molasses, honey, and candy.

Avoiding this type of sugar completely is very difficult, if not impossible. However, with dedication and education, many of my patients have made constructive changes to their diets.

Overall, reducing "added sugars" and selecting complex carbohydrates (as opposed to simple carbohydrates) as part of a balanced diet is most important. Complex carbohydrates are defined as large chains of sugar units arranged to form starches and fiber. These include vegetables, whole fruits, grains (brown rice, buckwheat, quinoa, oats, wheat, barley, corn), and legumes (chick peas, black-eyed peas, lentils, as well as beans such as lima, kidney, pinto, soy, and black beans). Starchy foods like pasta and white rice break down quickly to sugar and thus should be minimized.

When educating my patients and their caregivers, I tend to pass on the advice of a great scholar who taught me several things prior to medical school—my mother. "Everything in moderation" is what she emphasized. When making changes to one's diet, old habits are hard to break. This is especially true for patients with AD, who tend to crave sweets as the disease progresses. In my clinical practice, I am more insistent on these types of dietary modifications with a patient in the earlier stages of the disease, although there is the likelihood that dietary modifications across all stages are an important treatment intervention. In addition, I will occasionally advocate for the "early-bird" special technique when it comes to dietary modification. Prior to my family moving from New York to South Florida in 1997, I didn't understand much about the "early-bird" special. To explain further, there were several restaurants that offered special pricing deals when eating dinner before 6 pm. Not only can you save some money, but there may also be a brain-boosting effect of this strategy! In some patients, and only when approved by their primary care physician, waiting at least 12 hours in between dinner and breakfast can bring about a very mild state of "ketosis." This technique, combined with minimal (if any) carbohydrates in the morning, requires further research, but may make sense from a brain/body metabolism perspective.

Following a low-carbohydrate diet is not easy and is often easier said than done. For many patients with AD, eating balanced meals is enough of a challenge, and limiting food intake solely to the strategies listed here may not be feasible. Some of my most motivated patients and caregivers have made an honest attempt to strictly follow these recommendations, but have been unsuccessful. The decision on how closely one should try to follow these suggestions should be discussed in detail with the treating physician. If compliance is an issue, I remind my patients and caregivers that "it is what it is" and that it should not be a source of unnecessary frustration. Even following these suggestions a few days per week, or intermittently, may be better than not following them at all. Another important aspect is that patients with AD may have other co-existing medical diagnoses, and the dietary changes suggested here may not be applicable to those conditions. An evaluation by a competent medical professional, and even a dietician, may help to clarify these concerns.

A recent study by Dr. Craft and colleagues compared two different types of dietary interventions on cognitive outcomes: A Western-style diet (consisting of high saturated fat and high sugar) vs. an alternative Mediterranean-style diet (consisting of low saturated fat and low glycemic index carbohydrates).

Patients were divided into two groups:

Group 1:
Fat: 45% (25% of which saturated)
Carbohydrates: 35–40% (high glycemic index)
Protein: 15–20%

versus

Group 2:
Fat: 25% (<7% of which saturated)
Carbohydrates: 55–60% (low glycemic index)
Protein: 20–25%

The results of this study were quite interesting. The patients assigned to Group 2 (low fat, low sugar) did better in terms of memory function. There was a significant effect of diet on delayed memory. It was hypothesized that the low-fat diet improved memory possibly due to positive effects on inflammation, oxidative stress, insulin, and amyloid beta protein. In June 2011, Craft and colleagues published a fascinating paper (*Archives of Neurology*) supporting that "consumption of a diet high in saturated fat and simple carbohydrates may contribute to pathologic processes in the brain that increase the risk of Alzheimer's disease, while a diet low in saturated fat and simple carbohydrates may offer protection against dementia and enhance brain health." Further scientific research on diet and nutrition in AD is warranted.

Related to dietary changes, it is essential to avoid being overweight. Patients with Alzheimer's disease should be encouraged to become educated about nutrition and lose weight via a structured intervention program incorporating both diet and exercise, supervised by the treating physician.

How is obesity related to cognition? Increased body-mass index (BMI) and increased waist-to-hip ratio are linked to hippocampal volume in later life. Also, having high central adiposity (also known as a big stomach or a "big gut") increases risk of cognitive impairment (Whitmer and Yaffe, *Neurology* 2008).

Metabolic syndrome is a constellation of vascular risk factors that includes increased waist circumference, low HDL cholesterol, high triglycerides, high blood pressure, and abnormally elevated fasting blood glucose. Metabolic syndrome and obesity are both associated with accelerated cognitive aging, especially among those individuals with other medical illnesses that cause inflammation in the body.

Considering the information presented above, some believe that adopting a Mediterranean-style diet may be helpful for patients with AD. Fruits and vegetables, lean protein (fish, chicken, turkey), low-fat foods (especially low in saturated fats), nuts, and seeds are a part of this type of diet. Some advocate for minimizing consumption of red meat (no more than 1–2 times per week) and also minimizing the amount of processed foods in the diet.

When it comes to dietary choices, here are two good rules of thumb:

1. The fewer ingredients listed on the nutrition label—the better! (Suggestion courtesy of Cheryl Fawn.)

2. When eating dairy products, consider low-fat (or better yet, non-fat) options when possible.

We have talked about the importance of "good fat," or unsaturated fat, vs. "bad fat," or saturated and trans fats. It is important for patients and caregivers to learn the difference and make a habit of reading nutrition labels. In fact, it is important to read the "Nutrition Facts" information and ingredient list on foods when available, as this will help keep track of exactly what is put into the body, which has an effect on brain health.

While taking supplements, capsules, liquids, etc. that contain omega-3 fatty acids, more DHA than EPA is most important. Eating fish that are high in DHA and EPA is also advisable. There are several specific types of fish including mackerel, lake trout, herring, sardines, albacore tuna, and wild salmon that are high in these two kinds of omega-3 fatty acids. Tofu and other forms of soybeans may be helpful, as well as canola, walnut, and their oils. I advocate for patients to eat fish in moderation, roughly twice a week, to ensure a good supply of DHA and EPA while mitigating the potential for increasing mercury in the diet. The types of fish selected are also important (e.g., if the fish is farm-raised rather than wild-caught, the level of omega-3s may be significantly less).

Antioxidants in the diet are also very important. There are ongoing studies to determine whether eating a diet rich in antioxidants is helpful for cognition. Considering the risk-benefit ratio, I do tend to recommend incorporating antioxidant-rich foods into the diet. One study is looking at the combination of omega-3 fatty acids plus blueberry powder. The investigators will be capturing data on metabolic parameters, inflammation, and uptake of omega-3 fatty acids, as well as the effects on cognition.

There are several antioxidant-rich foods aside from blueberries that I recommend. These include several types of berries (e.g., raspberries, cranberries, acai, cherries, strawberries, blackberries, and elderberries). Other fruits like tomatoes (try heating them as this may increase the availability of the antioxidants to the body), pomegranates, red grapes (and grape juice), oranges, grapefruits, and apples are also high in antioxidants. I suggest at least a 1–2 servings per day.

There are a variety of vegetables that are high in substances that may protect the brain. These include carrots, broccoli, beets, spinach, kale, cabbage, Brussels sprouts, artichokes, collard, and other dark leafy greens. Other high-antioxidant foods include walnuts, pecans, dark chocolate, teas (green and black), and coffee (we will cover this in greater detail later).

Another recent study in animals looked at the combination of a diet high in antioxidants together with behavioral enrichment. Researchers have studied these interventions in dogs (beagles) since older animals develop a syndrome that is similar to Alzheimer's disease in humans. Dogs that develop cognitive deficits in middle age may be diagnosed with something commonly known as "Doggie Alzheimer's" or the more official term, canine cognitive dysfunction syndrome. These dogs give scientists a model that is similar to AD (but not exactly the same), as dogs demonstrate beta-amyloid in the brain with age, but no neural fiber networks of Tau protein (humans have both). Cognitive tests in dogs can be performed to help assess the effectiveness of an intervention, and their brains can be looked at under a microscope to determine if there are any effects apparent in the brain cells.

One study in dogs (beagles) over three years looked at whether dietary antioxidants would reduce oxidative damage. The antioxidant diet had vitamin E and C, as well as spinach, carrots, tomatoes, citrus, grapes, lipoic acid, and l-carnitine (supplements which may help to protect the mito- chondria). In addition to the enriched diet, dogs also participated in group exercise including three times per week of walking and running with other dogs (to incorporate socialization). Dr. Carl Cot- man and colleagues at the University of California at Irvine found that by the second year of the study, it was apparent that the intervention was working. By year three, the treatment group (diet and exer- cise) maintained cognition while almost 80% of the dogs that did not have the antioxidant-rich diet and exercise (control group) could no longer maintain the ability to perform specific cognitive tasks. In fact, over time the diet and exercise group dogs regained the capacity to perform a task that they could do when they were younger. The control group dogs were unable to relearn the task.

On a neurobiological or brain cell level, the treatment group demonstrated less oxidative dam- age to the part of the cell called the mitochondria and an increase in efficiency of the respiratory chain. Increased antioxidant defense enzymes were also apparent, which correlated with cognitive test results. BDNF, or brain-derived neurotrophic factor, was also most pronounced in the treatment group and approached the levels in younger animals. An article in the *Journal of Neuroscience* looked at amyloid protein load, which also decreased.

The take-home point here is that the combined treatment of an antioxidant-rich diet plus exercise led to improved mitochondrial function and better enabled protective mechanisms in the brain. While these studies need to be replicated in humans, it seems that exercise and behavioral enrichment synergize with diet to enhance brain health.

As such, in my clinical practice I advocate for these changes to be made by my AD patients, and I also suggest integrating socialization elements into their exercise routines. These "social" aspects may prove to be an important aspect toward maximizing brain health. Again, translating these findings to humans is necessary and will take several years, but why wait? Considering the risk-benefit ratio, this is a strategy that I consider for my patients.

While some clinicians advocate for taking vitamins in pill form, a balanced diet should provide most of the daily vitamin requirements. Ensuring adequate intake of vitamins such as folic acid and B_{12} are important, as is vitamin D.

Several studies have shown that a significant proportion of people are deficient in vitamin D, and that supplementation may be beneficial for brain protection. As such, I have recently started to consider adding 1,000–2,000 I.U. (or more) of vitamin D in pill form, along with at least 10–15 minutes of sunlight per day. The exact dose of vitamin D is unclear at this time. Due to this uncertainty (e.g., dose, whether or not a blood level should be drawn), the decision to take vitamins and in what amounts should always be discussed with and approved by the patient's primary care physician.

There has been a lot of discussion in the media about whether caffeine and coffee should be considered in the treatment plan of AD. While there are no scientific studies that specifically address this as a treatment for AD, I again use my mom's rule of "everything in moderation." A few cups earlier in the day are probably okay, as long as this has been approved by the treating physician. Caffeine may have effects on the heart (such as increasing heart rate) and may also increase anxiety. The most recent study in mice yielded some very interesting results. Cao and colleagues found that mice with Alzheimer's that drank the human equivalent of several cups of coffee each day had cognitive benefits (*Journal of Alzheimer's Disease*, June 2011). In addition, several studies (mostly in Europe) have shown the potential for a "protective" effect of caffeine/coffee on the brain.

To summarize, in my clinical practice I suggest focusing on these general categories of diet and nutrition in my patient population. When making such dietary changes, it may be helpful to keep a diet journal and meal log in order to keep track of what is eaten. It is also advisable to have laboratory studies (blood work) done before making dietary changes, as well as several weeks or months afterwards. Again, any and all changes should be under the guidance and supervision of the treating healthcare provider (e.g., physician, dietician).

TOP TEN DIET AND NUTRITION RECOMMENDATIONS

1. Include the following suggested breakdown of macronutrients (modified from Craft study):

   - Fat: 25% (<7% of which saturated)

   - Carbohydrates: 30–45% (low glycemic index)

   - Protein: 25–35%

2. Minimize carbohydrates with a high glycemic index—especially added simple sugars, high fructose corn syrup, and corn syrup in general.

   It is unclear what the exact target number of total carbs should be per day, but some suggest 130 grams/day (low-carb diet). Others suggest less than half that amount (very low-carbohydrate/ketogenic diet). Decrease dietary carbs slowly over weeks and with supervision and approval by a physician (see sample plan to follow). Patients with diabetes should avoid ketogenic diets as severe health consequences may occur.

3. Try a Mediterranean-style diet, including fruits

and vegetables, lean protein (fish, chicken, turkey), low-fat items, nuts, and seeds. Avoid excessive red meat intake as well as processed foods.

4. "Good" fat (unsaturated) vs. "bad" fat (saturated and trans fats)—learn the difference and avoid the "bad" fats!

5. Omega-3 fatty acids (DHA and EPA).

6. Antioxidants.

7. Vitamins: folic acid, B_{12}, vitamin D (via adequate nutrition, or supplement as needed in pill or liquid form).

8. In general, the fewer ingredients listed on the label, the better!

9. Low-fat (or non-fat) dairy products when possible.

10. Coffee (caffeinated): a few small cups earlier in the day are probably okay.

Regarding recommendation #2 above, I suggest the following step-wise approach toward dietary enhancement. Since there are potential negative health consequences of the diet plan below (as a patient's medical history needs to be considered before making such recommendations), any and all changes in diet need to be supervised and approved by the treating physician.

For example, patients with diabetes who are predisposed to a condition called ketoacidosis should not follow the diet below. Other potential side effects that have been reported from low-carbohydrate diets include constipation or diarrhea, headaches, and muscle weakness.

Week 1

DO NOT make any drastic changes to the diet. During the first week patients should become more "mindful" of what they are eating, look closer at nutrition labels and ingredients, and go food shopping at a variety of grocery and health food stores. This should help with education regarding what types of foods may be most favorable to eat. Read and re-read the recommendations above and below several times, and compare the food choices that have been made in the past with the choices planned for the future. Buy a scale (with a body fat analyzer) and begin a weekly log of weight, percent body fat, waist circumference, and activity level (include number of exercise sessions per week and total amount of exercise time). Record this information on diet journal log sheets found at www.TheADplan.com, and include all meals for two days during the week (e.g., Wednesday and Saturday).

Week 2

Continue diet log sheets as instructed above, and keep track of total grams of carbohydrates as best as possible. A variety of websites and handbooks can give estimates. Once approved by and only under close supervision of a physician, try for a goal of 130–150 grams of carbohydrates per day, and minimize those with a high glycemic index. Begin efforts to follow the general breakdown of macronutrients per day as described above (protein vs. fat vs. carbohydrates) and increase lean meats and low-fat options, while decreasing simple and added sugars. Try to eat fish at least twice this week and increase fruits, vegetables, and other foods rich in antioxidants.

Weeks 3–4

Continue diet log sheets as instructed above. Keep track of total grams of carbohydrates as best as possible, and now try for a goal of 110–130 grams of carbohydrates per day. Minimize those carbohydrates with a high glycemic index. Follow the general breakdown of macronutrients per day above (protein vs. fat vs. carbohydrates). Continue a stepwise increase in lean meats and low-fat options, while decreasing simple and added sugars. Try to eat fish at least two to three times per week, continue to increase foods rich in antioxidants, and increase fruits and vegetables.

Weeks 5–6

Continue as above but now try to decrease carbohydrates to 90–110 grams per day. Minimize those with a high glycemic index.

Weeks 7–8

Continue as above but now try to decrease carbs to 70–90 grams per day. Minimize those with a high glycemic index. If symptoms of ketoacidosis occur (Early signs: increasing fatigue, weakness, increased thirst, frequent urination, dry skin and tongue, leg cramps, fruity odor to the breath, upset stomach, nausea. Later signs: vomiting, shortness of breath, increased breathing rate or pulse), increase the amount of carbohydrates in the diet, and speak with the primary care doctor/treating physician. If symptoms are moderate or severe, go to the emergency room or see the primary care doctor or supervising physician immediately.

Week 9 and beyond

Continue diet as tolerated. Decrease carbs to 65 grams or less per day if tolerated. If symptoms of ketoacidosis occur (Early signs: increasing fatigue, tired and sleepy, weakness, increased thirst, frequent urination, dry skin and tongue, leg cramps, fruity odor to the breath, upset stomach, nausea.

Later signs: vomiting, shortness of breath, increased breathing rate or pulse), increase the amount of carbohydrates, and speak with the primary care doctor/treating physician. If symptoms are moderate or severe, go to the emergency room or see the primary care doctor or supervising physician immediately.

<hr>

While it may be necessary to have even fewer carbs than the amounts detailed above, any attempt at a very low-carbohydrate (ketogenic) diet must be made under the close supervision of a treating physician. In addition, using the combination of a ketogenic diet plus Axona may lead to severe consequences (e.g., ketoacidosis).

11. How often should an Alzheimer's patient be seen by a physician and what medical illnesses may increase the rate of cognitive decline?

Ongoing follow-up with the patient's primary care physician, and/or specialist is imperative for routine health maintenance. Any vascular risk factors (high blood pressure, cholesterol, diabetes/high blood sugars, etc.) have the potential to increase the rate of progression of memory decline.

Patients should have cholesterol results checked on a regular basis and consider treatment if levels are abnormal. Cholesterol drugs, also known as statin medications, may provide benefits in patients with high cholesterol. A recent study by Sano and colleagues in mild to moderate AD patients with normal cholesterol failed to show benefit of disease progression (*Neurology*, 2011). The risks and benefits of statin use should be discussed in detail with the physician. With my patients, I suggest statin

therapy in patients with borderline or high cholesterol. The treating physician must assess and
discuss with the patient and family about the risk-
benefit ratio of this type of therapy.

If an AD patient is treated solely by a primary
care physician (this may include an internal medicine or family medicine doctor), follow-up is suggested at a minimum of every four to six months
(two or three visits per year). If an AD patient is
also seeing a specialist (this may include a neurologist or psychiatrist), follow-up should occur at
a minimum of every six months, and one helpful
strategy would be to have four visits per year (once
every three months alternating primary care and
specialist appointments).

It is imperative that patients visit their physician
if symptoms worsen or change, or if new symptoms
or problems arise. In these situations, visits may
need to increase in frequency.

Another aspect about patient outcomes in Alzheimer's is that simultaneous medical illnesses will
affect memory and thinking skills in a negative way.
For example, a variety of studies show that inflammation and/or infections in the body may cause

increased inflammation in the hippocampus (Maier and colleagues, U. Colorado at Boulder). This is especially pronounced in older individuals, even without Alzheimer's disease. Additional medical conditions thought to affect cognition include surgeries, sleep disorders, and cancer, among a myriad of other diseases. In animal models, the effect of anesthesia during surgery has been studied. Some of these studies have found that the negative effects of anesthesia may be more related to the inflammatory processes during the surgery and not the anesthesia itself. Other scientists do not agree and feel that anesthesia itself may cause some deleterious effects.

12. How can the behavioral changes and psychiatric symptoms of Alzheimer's be best managed?

One of the most troubling aspects of Alzheimer's disease are changes in behavior, including anxiety, aggression, and depression. There are several strategies to help manage these types of symptoms.

Scientific studies suggest that in general, treating patients with the cholinesterase inhibitor medications (Aricept, Exelon, Razadyne ER) and memantine (Namenda) may be helpful for the behavioral aspects of AD. If behavioral troubles occur or worsen, patients must be evaluated by a qualified medical professional to ensure that the symptoms are not due to another treatable medical condition, such as a urinary tract infection, other infection, medication side effect, other medical illness, or a variety of other conditions. Most of the time when my patients call me with a sudden worsening or with acute changes in behavior, the cause is later attributed to a medical illness, as opposed to worsening of the Alzheimer's disease itself. Once the medical condition is treated, it may take several days or weeks for the patient to return back to their usual behavior and baseline cognitive functioning. Sometimes, despite the resolution of the medical illness, patients will not go back to the same cognitive baseline they were functioning at beforehand.

Once a thorough evaluation is completed, and all other medical or other causes aside from progression of Alzheimer's disease have been excluded, some practitioners may consider adding additional medications. The first medication class that I consider in my practice is the selective serotonin reuptake inhibitors, or SSRIs. These may obviate the need for antipsychotic medications, which may have more serious side effects. While there is no FDA-approval for the use of SSRIs for management of behavioral symptoms of AD, several clinicians have had success with agents such as citalopram (Celexa), escitalopram (Lexapro), and sertraline (Zoloft). There is some evidence that SSRIs may improve anxiety in older adults, but further study is necessary to determine their effect on anxiety in patients with AD. A recent study by Drs. Nelson and Devanand looked at seven studies of patients with depression and dementia (*Journal of the American Geriatric Society*, 2011). They found that there was some benefit of antidepressants, but this did not meet a "statistically significant" difference between drug- vs. placebo-treated patients. The authors noted that one problem with their findings was that all but one of the studies were small (less than 50 patients), and the trials may not have had enough patients enrolled to detect these statistical differences. They also noted that the variability in depression diagnoses, treatments used, and other patient characteristics may have also affected the results. Certain SSRI medications have been shown in animal models to have the potential for "neuroprotection," meaning there is the chance that they may slow down the progression of the disease. In addition to possibly reducing the need for stronger behavioral medications that have the potential for side effects, these SSRI medications have a generally favorable risk-benefit ratio and are relatively safe. As such, SSRIs (mainly citalopram) have been adjunctively used in my clinical practice.

Looking to the future, there is an ongoing trial called "CITAD" (began in 2008, to end in 2013, with results to follow) that aims to directly study the effect of citalopram in the treatment of AD.

Antipsychotic drugs may be recommended and must be used with strict supervision by a qualified medical professional. If necessary, in my clinical practice I tend to use the medication quetiapine (Seroquel) starting with very low doses in the evening, increasing very slowly and gradually. Risks and benefits of these medications must be discussed in detail between the physician, patient, and caregivers. It is important to note that the FDA has given antipsychotics a "black box" warning (printed in the PI of the drug), meaning that there may be specific dangers with using these medications in AD patients. This warning states that "elderly patients with dementia-related psychosis treated with antipsychotic drugs are at an increased risk of death." This data comes from several trials that show that use of these drugs increases the risk of death by approximately 1.6 times, most often due to heart problems or infection.

After reading that warning, readers may ask

why I have used these medications on numerous occasions for AD patients with severe behavioral issues (e.g., agitation, aggression, psychosis). The answer is that we have no other medications that have been proven to work. If my AD patient is already on, for example, Aricept (or Exelon), Namenda, and Celexa, and the behaviors are such that the patient is physically harming the caregiver or severe enough to require placement in a nursing home, families will often accept the risk-benefit ratio in order to protect the caregiver, keep the patient at home, and improve quality of life for the patient and the caregivers.

Aside from Seroquel, in my practice I have used several other medications in this class, but each has its own set of side effects on top of the black-box warning. There have been a few trials that have shown improvements in behavioral disturbances (e.g., agitation) and psychotic symptoms due to dementia in the elderly, but each drug may have adverse effects. As such, it is important to discuss these options closely with the prescribing physician.

Some physicians have seen benefit from the drug divalproex (Valproic Acid) for behavioral symptoms.

However, in addition to having the potential for side effects, one recent study by Tariot and colleagues found that this drug did not delay emergence of agitation or psychosis (*Archives of General Psychiatry*, 2011), and another study by Fleisher and colleagues showed a greater loss in brain size, and a more rapid decline on one commonly used cognitive test, but not on others (*Neurology*, September 2011).

There are also several non-pharmacologic interventions that may be helpful (Cohen-Mansfield, 1995). These include environmental interventions such as:

- Behavioral therapies

- Structured activities

- Sensory intervention

- Social contact or simulated interaction

- Light therapy

- Hearing aids

- Pain management

- Caregiver/staff training

13. What are some options for treating AD patients who have difficulty falling asleep at night?

There are several options to treat sleep difficulties. However, there is one specific medication that I tend to use more than others. In addition, one of the strategies that I try to use is to avoid sedative medications in the category called benzodiazepines, commonly known as diazepam (Valium), lorazepam (Ativan), and clonazepam (Klonopin), as well as similar medications such as zolpidem (Ambien). In my clinical practice, I prefer using a medication like trazodone (Desyrel) at low doses before bedtime. This medication needs to be used under the supervision of a qualified medical professional.

I always use the strategy of "start low, go slow" when using these medications. For trazodone, I will most commonly start with 25 mg about 30 minutes before bedtime (sometimes starting lower at 12.5 mg, especially in my oldest patients). I try to use this dose for at least a few days or up to a week before making an increase. If the medication is not helpful after a week or so, I will increase to 50 mg before bedtime, as tolerated. I will continue to reassess every week, but try to avoid using more than a maximum of 100 or 150 mg at night. Usually 50, 75, or 100 mg is the highest dose that I prescribe in my patients, although this is quite variable depending upon the patient and severity of disease.

Other agents that may be considered include eszopiclone (Lunesta) and ramelton (Rozerem). Some clinicians use Lunesta with caution as it is also a benzodiazepine receptor agonist and has a longer half-life, possibly worsening the "hangover effect" on cognition in the morning. A renowned sleep specialist that I have worked with utilizes mirtazapine (Remeron) instead, which can help sleep at low doses of 7.5mg each evening. At low doses, Remeron is generally well tolerated but at higher doses, adverse effects may occur (e.g., weight gain).

Daytime bright light exposure is postulated to strengthen (increase the amplitude) of the circadian (biological-clock driven) sleep-wake rhythm. This is also a helpful recommendation that may be considered.

14. What other general recommendations may be helpful for either the patient or the caregiver?

Caregiver support is essential. If the stress and fatigue of being a caregiver begins to affect his or her own health and well-being, not soon after will the patient's condition also decline. I advocate for a social worker to get involved early, and I spend a great deal of time with patients to make sure that the caregiver has adequate support. I also emphasize quite strongly something that I learned from my cousin Cynthia, who did an amazing and admirable job caring for my uncle Bob. I try to convey to caregivers that it is okay to let people help. Taking periodic breaks is essential as it helps to keep up one's strength so they can do more for their loved one later. Some other activities that she taught me that loved ones can do together are folding laundry (especially mixing and matching socks), brushing the dog, and collecting shells on the beach. As time progresses, additional individual and group activities can be found to both help the caregiver and give them a well-deserved break.

I commonly suggest reaching out to the Alzheimer's Association (www.alz.org) as an initial contact. Early and continued caregiver support is essential. I also suggest an evaluation by a licensed clinical social worker, therapist, or geriatric care manager who can help give advice, support, do a home assessment, etc. They can also suggest activity programs within the community and other available resources such as adult daycare and activity programs (when necessary). There is an excellent book on this subject that I recommend to my patients by Nataly Rubinstein MSW, LCSW, C-ASWCM, *Alzheimer's Disease and Other Dementias: The Caregiver's Complete Survival Guide*. I also consider a home health assessment and visiting nurse referral to help with medication management across all stages of the disease, especially if there are recent medication changes or if the patient or caregiver is having trouble keeping up with medication management.

There are a variety of support groups all across

the country. Each year there are a multitude of educational programs and conferences sponsored by the Alzheimer's Association and other organizations for patients, caregivers, and family members. Try contacting the local chapter by phone or review their website. See the Resources section at the end of the book for information on memory disorders centers throughout the United States.

There are several other helpful hints that I recommend. Bringing family members to every physician appointment is essential. Any patient with cognitive impairment of any degree (from the most mild to most severe) should always be accompanied by at least one, better yet two or three family members or friends. Family members or friends can provide historical details of the memory complaints and day-to-day functioning that are essential for the physician to form an optimized management plan. In addition, having one person take notes or ask specific questions (written down prior to the appointment) will help with the overall care plan and possibly patient outcomes. Believe it or not, most physicians appreciate patient and caregiver questions! Developing a long-term partnership with the physician and staying educated and informed are essential in AD care.

Due to changes in the healthcare system and provider reimbursement, many physicians are often struggling to make ends meet. If you are fortunate to have found a physician who spends valuable time with you in developing this partnership, don't forget to thank them and the office staff for their kindness and help!

15. Why do some of these interventions work well in select patients and not work well in others?

We are learning more about the answer to this question with each year that passes. One of the most important areas where we still need to learn more about is genetics. Depending on their genetic code, or DNA, patients may tend to respond better to one treatment versus another, or may not respond at all.

This field, called pharmacogenomics, is rapidly expanding but a detailed explanation is beyond the scope of this book. In short, we now know that having one copy of the APOE4 gene may decrease the chances of responding to several therapies. In fact, certain treatments like DHA fish oil, Axona (medical food), and a vaccine that is currently being studied called bapineuzumab have shown that patients with certain genes respond better than others without that type of genetic code. Much research needs to be done to clarify these points, and we are not yet at the point where most practitioners would send blood samples for DNA typing in order to make treatment decisions. If you are a healthcare professional reading this book, I would suggest reading our article on Genetics of Dementia in the *Continuum* series (American Academy of Neurology, April 2011) for more detailed information.

There are also a number of studies about the power of positive thinking. In other words, if the patient or caregiver, or even the physician, "thinks" a medication or other treatment will work, it might actually have a higher likelihood of working in certain medical conditions. I strongly believe that maintaining a positive attitude is extremely important for both patients and caregivers throughout the entire duration of the disease. Remember this important quote: "Think positive, and it will be positive!"

16. Why hasn't my doctor recommended several of the options mentioned in this book?

Many of the patients who are referred to me for a second opinion have not been instructed by their physician to begin several of the treatments mentioned here. This does not mean that the referring physician is doing anything wrong. In fact, if the treating physician is going "by the book" and following FDA guidelines, a patient with mild to moderate dementia of the Alzheimer's type should be taking only one medication, and a patient with moderate to severe disease should be taking two medications together.

As I said before, and for several reasons, I prefer a much more comprehensive approach to the treatment of this disease. As long as there is some evidence or potential for effectiveness and the interventions are generally safe, I believe that the risk-benefit ratio of multimodal therapy favors the comprehensive approach detailed in this text.

Some physicians remain skeptical of any treatment or intervention that is not FDA-approved. I understand their concerns but again, I treat all patients as if they were my own family members and would rather try these treatments, which are relatively safe, than not try them at all.

Some physicians do not feel that based on the evidence available, treating even with the FDA-approved medications is warranted. I have discussed this topic with several well-known and well-trained physicians. They base their decisions on the results of research trials, the potential for side effects, and the cost of the medications.

I respectfully disagree with this approach. I feel that the patient sitting in front of me is an individual. In my opinion, making treatment decisions based on the results of large studies that focus on large numbers of patients is quite helpful and very important, but it is only one piece of the puzzle. I take a comprehensive approach to AD and feel that giving several options with a favorable risk-benefit ratio is preferable.

For example, one way to look at the use of

cholinesterase inhibitor medications is to generalize the response rates. Some clinicians feel that when a patient is started on a cholinesterase inhibitor, there is roughly a 33% chance that the patient will improve, a 33% chance that the patient will stabilize, and a 33% chance that the patient will continue to decline with no benefit at all. Some physicians would say that "only" having a 33% chance of improvement, combined with the cost and potential for side effects (e.g., nausea, vomiting, diarrhea, or even cardiac rhythm problems like a slowed heartbeat) would deter their recommendation of using that drug in their patients.

Again, I respectfully disagree. Even if there is "only" a 33% chance of improvement, 33% is much higher than zero percent! In addition, based on one small randomized, double-blinded, placebo-controlled study, adding folic acid 1 mg in combination with the cholinesterase inhibitor could increase the positive response rate from about 39% to 70%.

A variety of studies have also shown that when cholinesterase medications are withheld, there is a decline in cognitive function (when compared with treatment) after only six months. In my practice, since I never know which patient may respond, I almost always offer treatment as an option to my patients.

17. With all of these options to treat AD, where should we begin?

It is very important to begin any new therapies in a slow and step-wise manner. It is a good general rule to always start only one new intervention (medication, supplement, medical food) at a time. For some drugs, supplements, or medical foods, a slow start (initially using the lowest dose with incremental increases over time) may reduce the likelihood of side effects. Also, when starting more than one treatment at the same time, it may be impossible to know which one caused a side effect if one were to occur.

The decision of when to start the aforementioned therapies and in what combination is quite complex and must be made by a qualified medical professional who will be treating the patient on an ongoing basis. When a patient is first diagnosed with mild Alzheimer's, I usually start a cholinesterase inhibitor first in combination with 1 mg of folic acid each day. After slowly increasing the dose of the cholinesterase inhibitor, and once it is well tolerated and stable, I may then suggest DHA fish oil with slow increases, followed by adding curcumin 3–4 weeks later. The medical food Axona may also be considered once the above therapies are well tolerated. Once the disease begins to progress, or even at times somewhat earlier, I will consider using Namenda. If problems with attention, depression, or other mild behavioral complaints occur, I may consider citalopram (Celexa).

As soon as the diagnosis of AD is suspected, several non-pharmacologic interventions should be implemented, including physical and mental exercise, a music activity program, dietary changes, and other lifestyle modifications.

18. Are there any treatments that you do not recommend or whose effectiveness you are unsure of?

There are several treatments that have been thought of in the past as helpful, but currently, considering the most recent scientific evidence, these treatments have fallen out of favor. I do not recommend high-dose vitamin E (no more than 400–800 I.U. per day) as some studies have shown potential risk (especially in patients with cardiac disease). I do not recommend ginkgo biloba, as evidence is lacking for treatment, and there is the potential for side effects. There is also a large study on ginkgo biloba that showed no benefit toward prevention. There are several other treatments where the scientific data is still unclear, so at this time, I do not incorporate them into my clinical management. Interested individuals can read about a variety of potential treatments on the Internet or find several supplements and vitamins in the health food store that claim to have a "brain-boosting" effect. However, at the time of publication, I limit patient recommendations to those detailed in this book.

19. Where can I turn to for help, should I get a second opinion, and how can I learn more about ongoing research studies that I can participate in?

There are a variety of ways to get help, and one of the best options is the Alzheimer's Association. They have a 24-hour helpline that can answer a variety of questions (1-800-272-3900) as well as give some general recommendations of services in the area. Their website is also quite helpful: www.alz.org. The Alzheimer's Foundation of America (www.alzfdn.org) also provides support and educational resources for patients and care-givers. Many communities may also have additional organizations that can help on a local level, so be sure to ask around and search on the Internet.

Another resource is the Alzheimer's Disease Education and Referral Center, which can help educate on AD as well as provide referrals for clin-ical research studies and other information. Their phone number is 1-800-438-4380 and website is www.nia.nih.gov/alzheimers.

In regard to a second opinion, seeing another physician with specialty training in AD may be helpful. If an Alzheimer's specialist is not available in the local area, seeing either a neurologist or geriatric psychiatrist in addition to the primary care doctor is another option.

Throughout the country, there are several Alzheimer's Disease Research Centers that focus on clinical care and research. Some of the most well-known physicians are affiliated with these centers, although many of them primarily focus on research. If a patient is interested in getting involved in a research study (often referred to as a "clinical trial"), these centers may be an option.

Remember that at such academic centers, many clinicians practice "by the book" evidence-based medicine and may not recommend several of the options reviewed in this book. However, these centers have a variety of resources and special expertise that one may be looking for.

Aside from these centers, learning about doctors from other patients and caregivers has been one of the best strategies my patients have utilized. Going to caregiver support programs and other activities sponsored by the Alzheimer's Association, for example, may help to meet others who are satisfied with physicians practicing in the area.

The decision about whether or not to be evaluated for a clinical trial should be discussed in detail with the patient, family members, and treating physician. In my practice, roughly 20% of my patients are currently enrolled in a research study trying to determine the effectiveness of a new therapy for AD. A key consideration with almost all clinical trials is that a certain number of participants (usually 50%) will receive the investigational agent, and the rest of the patients will get a placebo, an inactive substance that should have no effect whatsoever. There are several ongoing clinical trials that have promise; however, we will not know the results until several months or even years after the trial is complete. To learn more about these, ask the treating physician or search on the Internet. There is a website sponsored by the U.S. Government (www.clinicaltrials.gov) that keeps a list of ongoing and recently completed research studies for thousands of diseases, including AD. The Alzheimer's Association has a website called TrialMatch™ (www.alz.org/trialmatch, phone 800-272-3900) that began in 2010. This service provides individualized matching services for patients with AD, mild cognitive impairment, and related dementias, as well as information for their caregivers, family members, and healthcare providers. Available studies are found based on several factors, including specific diagnosis, stage, treatment history, and location. The service is free and confidential. As of late 2011, the service listed over 130 research studies at over 500 sites across the country.

20. Can you summarize the most optimal treatment plan for AD?

When I lecture to clinicians all around the country, several ask me to share with them the recommendations that I make to my patients so that they can improve their patient care. I freely share these recommendations with allied health professionals, including physicians, nurses, nurse practitioners, physician assistants, and pharmacists.

This "recipe" is what I feel is the best way to treat AD. While I cannot guarantee that everything on this list will make a difference, I can 100% honestly say that this would be the exact treatment outline that I would consider for my own family member, and, of course, to patients in my practice. I learned from one of my past professors that patient care should not be based solely on an algorithm. This means that each patient should be considered on an individual basis. In other words, every patient should absolutely not follow this exact plan. Any treatment regimen must be carefully tailored for each individual patient by the treating physician, and closely supervised by the physician.

When I first developed and started sharing this plan in 2005, I called it my "Ten-Step Alzheimer's Plan." In 2006, the name changed to my "Twelve-Step Plan." Now, we are up to the "Twenty-Step Alzheimer's Plan." That statistic alone should be quite encouraging for anyone reading this book, as in only the last several years I have been able to *double* the number of recommendations that I make to patients!

Back when I started medical school, there were essentially no treatments for AD. In 2013, I hope that the name of my trusted plan changes again, and that in future years, we continue the great progress we have made thus far.

If I try to envision the future of Alzheimer's disease, there are several interventions on the horizon that generate excitement. There are a number of new and innovative therapies currently in trial. Some of the therapies include vaccine treatments and other medications that can be taken via a pill or intravenous (IV) therapy. Discussion of these treatments is beyond the scope of this book, as there is still much work to be done. I am confident that in the future, hopefully within the next 5 to 7 years, we will be making significant progress in the treatment of this disease.

As I have said time and time again at the end of every lecture I give on the topic of treating AD, there is no one "magic bullet" or "magic pill" for Alzheimer's. However, combination therapy following the steps listed in my 20-Step Plan for Alzheimer's Treatment (beginning on page 144) may yield the most benefit. Using these strategies, and with exciting advances on the way, there is more hope now than ever for patients with AD.

20-Step Plan for Alzheimer's Treatment

1. Exelon patch 4.6 mg each day for four weeks, then increase to 9.5 mg patch if tolerated. Place patch on the upper back (see picture in package insert) to clean, dry, hairless skin. Rotate application site each day to reduce possibility of irritation and make sure to take off the old patch before putting on a new one. The same exact spot should not be used within 14 days.

OR

Aricept 5 mg each day with food (breakfast or lunch, whichever meal is bigger). After four weeks, and only if tolerated, increase to 10 mg daily. After at least three months, consider Aricept 23 mg each day for severe patients (also must be taken with food and be careful to watch for side effects).

2. Folic acid 1 mg each day. Start with cholinesterase inhibitor.

3. Fish oil capsules, slowly increasing to at least three capsules each day. Must have DHA in it, the more the better (some EPA is okay as well). While the most recent study (*JAMA*) of algae-based DHA did not slow overall cognitive decline, benefit was seen in APOE4 negative patients, and other studies have shown benefit of fish oil derived from fish. Try to get at least 250 mg of DHA in each capsule for a total of at least 1,000–1,500 mg each day of DHA specifically. Try one capsule at first each day with a big meal and with water or juice, then increase if tolerated to twice per day. Consider Carlson Super DHA Gems, which have 500 mg of DHA and 200 mg of EPA per capsule. Another brand is Life's DHA (Martek), which may only work in APOE4 negative patients, but any brand with a high amount of DHA is suggested. (Fish oil capsules usually have 1,000 mg of *total* fish oil in each capsule, but each has a varied amount of actual DHA.) As an alternative to capsules, a liquid fish oil may be used. One brand to consider is called Nutri Supreme (available online at www.nutri-supreme.com or by calling 1-888-68-NUTRI), which is also kosher.

4. Once tolerating the above for a few months, consider Axona (medical food) half packet per day with food (preferably breakfast or lunch, whichever meal is bigger) for one week, then increase to 1 packet per day. First pour 6–8 oz of water, Boost/Ensure, skim milk, or other liquid into the shaker cup provided in the sample kit (or other shaker cup). Then add powder and shake/blend in order to improve tolerability. For at least the first few weeks, must take after a big meal and sip slowly over at least 20–30 minutes.

5. Curcumin (turmeric root). Buy in a health food store.

6. As disease progresses, consider adding memantine (Namenda) to cholinesterase inhibitor medication—increase this medication slowly to 10 mg twice a day (or Namenda XR 28 mg each day once released on the market).

7. Increase physical activity as tolerated and as approved by the primary care physician (PCP). Suggest personal trainer if motivation is a problem, as physical exercise improves brain function as well as benefiting the rest of the

body. Recommend exercise at least 3–4 times a week, for 45–60 minutes if tolerated.

8. Maintain a healthy diet (discuss with PCP or dietician) and stay in good physical health. Include fish like mackerel, lake trout, herring, sardines, albacore tuna, and wild salmon in the diet. These types of fish are high in two kinds of omega-3 fatty acids, eicosapentaenoic acid (EPA) and docosahexaenoic acid (DHA). Tofu and other forms of soybeans, canola, walnut, and their oils may be helpful as well. Anti-oxidants, fruits, vegetables, and lean meats are important. (See Chapter 10 for additional details about diet and nutrition strategies in Alzheimer's disease.)

9. Continue mental activity, including video games like Brain Age, Big Brain Academy, etc. (Nintendo DS or Nintendo Wii), puzzles, word games, reading books, crosswords, and other games requiring thought. Cognitive activities may be helpful a few times per week (challenging the brain may help maintain it), but some of the latest research has cautioned against excessive mental activities. The website www .lumosity.com is good for brain activities and

tracks patient progress (recommended use is once per week).

10. Listen to music (especially classical) and consider music activity programs including www .TherapyForMemory.com and other one-on-one therapy sessions.

11. Increase socialization, including activity programs, adult education classes, and social groups. Learning a new language, studying a new subject, or taking up new hobbies, especially in group settings, may be especially useful.

12. Ongoing follow-up with primary care physician for routine health maintenance. Any vascular risk factors (high blood pressure, cholesterol, high sugars, etc.) will increase the rate of progression of memory decline. Have cholesterol results checked and consider treatment. Risks and benefits of statin use should be discussed in detail. Consider ACE inhibitor (e.g., lisinopril, perindopril, or captopril due to their ability to cross the blood-brain barrier).

13. Consider adding vitamin D 1,000–2,000 I.U. (or more) each day. Risk-benefit ratio should be

discussed in detail with the patient and family. Consider approximately 10–15 minutes of sunlight per day, if approved by your treating physician.

14. Once on cholinesterase inhibitor and memantine, if behavioral troubles occur, consider using SSRI (e.g., citalopram) to obviate the need for anti psychotic medications. Avoid benzodiazepines, zolpidem (Ambien), etc.

15. Once on cholinesterase inhibitor and memantine, if sleep troubles occur, consider trazodone, ramelton (Rozerem), or eszopiclone (Lunesta). Avoid benzodiazepines, zolpidem (Ambien), etc.

16. Get a social worker involved early, and make sure caregiver has adequate support. Suggest Alzheimer's Association (www.alz.org) as an initial contact. Early and continued caregiver support is essential. Consider evaluation by a licensed clinical social worker who can help to give advice, be supportive, do a home assessment, etc. They can also suggest activity programs and a personal trainer, if desired. Join local support groups.

17. Consider home health assessment/visiting nurse referral to help with medication management.

18. Diet modification (see Chapter 10 for more details).

Recommendations for healthcare providers in evaluation/diagnosis:

19. If ordering a brain MRI, request thin cuts through the hippocampus/temporal lobe (e.g., MPRAGE sequence or epilepsy protocol, no contrast). Ask radiologist to assess for hippocampal atrophy, but it is most optimal for an experienced Alzheimer's clinician to review the actual films, when possible.

20. Consider neuropsychological testing. Neuropsychologists often make good recommendations based on the specific cognitive deficits that are identified.

21. Will I get Alzheimer's disease? Are my chances higher if I have a family member with AD?

I get this question quite frequently, but before I answer, let me clarify a few things. In general, Alzheimer's disease is a very common condition regardless of whether a person has a family member with the disease or not.

Let's summarize some of the general statistics. According to a recent National Institutes of Health report, one in seven people aged 71 and over will have dementia of any cause. The most common cause of dementia is Alzheimer's disease. By the age of 85, statistics show that over 40% of people will have Alzheimer's disease. Remember that these statistics are essentially irrespective of family history. The take-home point here is that everyone's risk for AD increases over time because the number-one risk factor is advancing age.

That being said, there are specific genes that can be passed on through generations that may increase the likelihood of developing Alzheimer's. The good news here is that only 6% of cases of AD are due to the types of genes that cause early-onset Alzheimer's. We won't get into detail here, but these genetic mutations include presenilin-1, presenilin-2, and amyloid precursor protein gene mutation. These genes contribute to the development of AD in patients younger than age 60.

There is another set of genes that is associated with older-age onset of AD, or late-onset Alzheimer's. The most well studied of these genes is called apolipoprotein epsilon-4 (or commonly referred to as APOE4). In summary, we all get one copy of the APOE gene from our mother, and another copy from our father. There are three types of these genes, APOE2, APOE3, and APOE4. If someone has one or more of the APOE4s, the risk of developing AD will increase. However, at the time of publication of this book, genetic testing for APOE is not recommended. Knowing whether a patient has one or more copies of APOE4 does not necessarily help a physician predict if or when a person will develop AD. Conversely, having one or more copies of APOE2 confers a reduced risk of developing AD.

We still have a long way to go in terms of using genetic testing to help with the pre-symptomatic diagnosis of AD. As such, in my practice I do not recommend genetic testing on family members of Alzheimer's patients, and instead suggest that all family members focus on a healthy lifestyle plan as detailed in the next few chapters.

Many experts feel that the rise in AD cases diagnosed in the last few decades is due to a variety of factors other than the advancing age of our population. One of these key considerations is the improved ability to make an accurate AD diagnosis.

Note that this would suggest that the incidence of AD has been much higher in previous years, but we are just now able to see this. With the advance of the medical field, doctors are now able identify patients with AD in a variety of ways, and hopefully in the future, we will be able to use biomarkers (like a blood test) to determine risk many years before the onset of symptoms. Other experts feel that based on the scientific evidence, one of the reasons that there has been an increase in the number of AD cases is the change in diet and nutrition patterns, particularly in the United States. Dr. Christopher Ochner (Columbia University College of Physicians and Surgeons) has pointed out to me on several occasions that portion sizes, average meal intake, adult obesity, and childhood obesity are critical issues that may also be related. Fast food on every corner, processed foods in every vending machine, and sugar, sugar, and more sugar added to just about anything and everything in arm's reach. People are eating more fat and fewer fruits and vegetables than ever before. This "Western diet" has been extensively studied and results show that this type of diet is associated with a higher risk of developing AD (more on this later). By now, many of us understand that sugar is "bad" when it comes to the well-known condition of diabetes. But what is not yet fully understood are the long- and short-term effects of carbohydrates (e.g., sugar) on Alzheimer's disease.

Whatever the reason for the explosion of AD cases, in my clinical practice, I consider "anything and everything, as long as it is safe." The following chapters will review the approach that I take for family members at risk of developing AD.

22. I have a family member with Alzheimer's and am concerned about developing AD. What strategies do you suggest for possible prevention?

Many of my suggestions are quite similar to some of the treatment interventions I employ for patients who have already been diagnosed with Alzheimer's. While not 100% proven by scientific studies, I believe that several of the strategies described in this section may be beneficial, in addition to having a favorable risk-benefit ratio.

While we will go into greater detail in the upcoming chapters, the take-home message about preventing or reducing the risk of developing AD is living a healthy lifestyle. Does exercise occur on a regular basis? It better! Smoking cigarettes? Stop! Significantly overweight? Lose weight! Been diagnosed with high blood pressure or high cholesterol? See a doctor and get treatment!

The effect of diet on the overall health of the

body starts early—in the womb! This means that the food a pregnant mother eats during pregnancy has an effect on future medical illnesses and control of weight. One study by Sinclair and colleagues (*Proceedings of the National Academy of Sciences*, 2007) showed that reductions in B_{12}, folate, and methionine from the maternal diet (in animals) increased adiposity (fat deposition), high blood pressure, insulin resistance, etc. in the offspring later in life.

We have made several advances in the understanding of cognitive changes with aging, most specifically Alzheimer's disease, but there is still work be done.

Just because one is getting older does not mean that he or she will automatically develop dementia! AD is not inevitable, but remember that there are some changes in cognition that occur "normally" with age. This condition is called age-associated cognitive impairment. Symptoms may include intermittent memory loss, word-finding difficulties, and slowing of the speed of thinking. When cognitive changes are isolated to difficulties with memory, this condition is sometimes referred to as age-related memory loss.

We also now know that while the brain does age over time, compensation also occurs. In other words, there is a rearrangement of function on multiple levels, from very small (e.g., brain cells and molecules) to very large (e.g., behaviors). It should be our goal to engage in certain activities and life behaviors during early and midlife (to be discussed), as these activities may improve one's ability to compensate for declining brain function later.

There are a variety of genetic and environmental risk factors for cognitive decline (e.g., Alzheimer's disease, age-associated cognitive decline). For example, the highest HDL cholesterol levels ("good" cholesterol) are associated with the most preserved thinking skills in individuals over 100 years old. In fact, there are several lifestyle factors (e.g., amounts of exercise and stress) and several medical conditions (e.g., vascular risk factors, metabolic syndrome, inflammation) that relate to changes in thinking skills and memory.

Most individuals who have risk factors for vascular disease suffer from "asymptomatic" vascular disease. In other words, there are no clinical symptoms that occur. However, even without any apparent symptoms, there is still "silent" damage that is occurring. With increasing age, a good portion of patients in their 80s have evidence of vascular disease in their brains, as seen on brain imaging. This theory links cognitive aging to an interaction of several coexisting diseases. Small, clinically silent strokes (death of tissue in the brain) are seen as bright "spots" on a brain scan commonly referred to as an MRI (magnetic resonance imaging). These are referred to as "white matter hyperintensities," which increase in prevalence and extent with age and have most recently been found to be associated with deficits in cognitive ability. Past and ongoing research by Drs. Au, DeCarli, and Wright will help elucidate these points in the future.

Healthy young adults are able to process information in their brain more efficiently than older adults with evidence of vascular damage (even when this damage was "clinically silent," meaning no symptoms or signs on neurological or cognitive evaluation). Another way of understanding this point is that older adults with vascular damage process information less efficiently than healthy young adults without vascular insults.

Aging in general is associated with cognitive decline and an increase in vascular risk. These vascular risks are associated with wider spread and more rapid decline of thinking skills and greater age differences in brain function.

Several models have been proposed that help us understand the variety of factors that affect memory and cognition. One study called the Northern Manhattan Study (Dr. Sacco and colleagues) has been researching environmental and genetic aspects of age-related cognitive changes, where patients have been followed for nearly 20 years. Based on this research, "successful" cognitive aging occurred in approximately 30% of patients. One way to help determine which patients will age successfully or have cognitive decline over time is by using a Global Vascular Risk Score. This score was developed as part of this study and takes into consideration markers such as obesity, blood pressure, exercise, and alcohol consumption. Many of these risk factors not only contributed to vascular damage in the brain, but also to shrinkage of the brain and the progression and/or onset of Alzheimer's. Using a combination of these factors, an online calculator has been developed to provide an estimate of risk of future health issues. Visit http://neurology.med.miami.edu/gvr/gvr.htm for more info (website is for research purposes only and does not provide medical advice).

While the discussion in this text focuses on strategies for avoiding or delaying the onset of Alzheimer's disease, it is possible that several of these suggestions may help to delay the onset of other causes of cognitive decline as well.

As one example, aerobic exercise reduces the shrinkage of the brain and also increases blood flow. Life stress can also lead to a variety of negative consequences, like impaired cognition in war veterans or impaired "episodic" memory in laboratory animals. A variety of medical diagnoses also contribute to memory loss or cognitive decline. One of the most common and fortunately treatable conditions is high blood pressure in midlife, which correlates with impaired thinking skills later in life. This is compared to research that shows that low blood pressure in late life may also lead to worse outcomes.

There is often considerable disagreement over defining what the "normal" or expected cognitive changes are that occur with age. We still have much to learn about the differences between Alzheimer's disease vs. "normal" age-related cognitive changes vs. other types of dementia, like vascular dementia.

Both young and older individuals use their hippocampus (memory center in the brain) as well as other neural networks that help to recall and remember things. The pathologic amyloid protein that accumulates in the brain of AD patients may be responsible for memory dysfunction, or may occur as a result of another process that causes the dysfunction. While this is the characteristic pathologic finding in AD, evidence of amyloid has been found in "normal" individuals at younger ages (up to one-third of normal individuals over the age of 65 have amyloid in their brain!). While it is not known whether these individuals will go on to develop AD, as there are no pre-symptomatic diagnostic tests at this time, anything that we can do to lower this amyloid protein may be beneficial before the onset of AD symptoms.

We also know that having a high level of "cognitive reserve" may improve outcomes when a cognitive disorder occurs in later life. Building this reserve, or "backup," begins at birth, accelerates during schooling, and continues throughout young and mid-adult life.

Researchers have studied IQ as a measure of cognitive reserve. It seems that patients with a high IQ have a less significant effect of amyloid on thinking skills and memory. This compares with individuals who have lower IQs that *do* tend to be affected by amyloid deposition.

Now, amyloid may not be the answer here, and there is some data that contradicts the comments above. Another study called the "90 plus study" looked at individuals 90 years of age and older (average age of 96). On average, one-third had dementia, one-third had cognitive impairment without dementia, and the rest were normal (Kawas, 2010). When they looked at the brains of the participants of this study, nearly 50% of the patients had amyloid in their brain. However, many of these individuals were cognitively normal.

In this study, determinants of successful aging in individuals over the age of 90 were related to several factors, including oxygenation, physical performance (hand grip, speed of walking), and blood pressure. It is not clear whether being on blood pressure medications was the cause of better cognition, or if having higher blood pressure increased blood flow to the brain. When blood pressure is taken, it is commonly reported as 120 over 70, or 120/70. The "top" number represents the systolic pressure, and the "bottom" number represents the diastolic pressure. While some studies have shown diastolic blood pressure may be more relevant, other studies have found the opposite. It appears that there is more research that needs to be done, especially in different populations with different ages, ethnic groups, and socioeconomic backgrounds.

Next, we will review the pharmacologic and non-pharmacologic interventions that may be utilized toward the possible prevention of AD.

23. Do you recommend the FDA-approved Alzheimer's drugs for prevention?

No. There is no evidence that using these medications in patients with no symptoms, or using these medications years in advance of the onset of symptoms, has any benefit for preventing Alzheimer's. I feel strongly that these medications should not be used for such purposes.

The Alzheimer's drugs like Aricept, Exelon patch, and Razadyne ER are indicated for mild to moderate AD. Again, there is no evidence showing that these medications prevent AD. However, while not FDA-approved, there is some evidence to suggest that patients with a diagnosis of mild cognitive impairment (MCI), most notably of the MCI-amnestic ("amnestic" meaning memory) form, may have some benefit of these drugs. MCI is commonly characterized by changes in cognition that have been identified by a physician, but these changes have not yet impacted the patient's activities of daily living. In my clinical experience, and based on the April 2011 AD diagnostic criteria discussed earlier, patients with MCI-amnestic may most commonly have "pre-Alzheimer's," or prodromal AD (at risk for developing AD). Patients in this category may derive benefit from the interventions discussed in this section and may even benefit from these FDA-approved drugs that would have to be prescribed "off-label" by a physician. That being said, I still do not feel that these medications are neuroprotective or preventative in the strict sense of the word. They may, however, help some of the cognitive symptoms associated with MCI.

24. Do you recommend any supplements or vitamins for prevention of Alzheimer's disease?

Yes. In my clinical practice, I suggest two supplements and several vitamins to possibly delay the onset of Alzheimer's disease.

Supplements

Fish oil has been studied in a variety of scientific trials, and there is evidence for its usefulness in Alzheimer's. There is some evidence that using specific types of fish oil may possibly delay the onset of the disease. The most recent trial that has been published was called MIDAS (November 2010), and we will discuss this study later in the chapter.

I want to clarify a few points about fish oil that I mentioned earlier in Section 2. There are different types of fish oil that are most commonly made up of omega-3 fatty acids and omega-6 fatty acids. While there is still much research to be done in order to determine what types work best, in my clinical practice I preferably recommend the omega-3s, mainly docosahexaenoic acid (DHA) and eicosapentaenoic acid (EPA). When visiting the supermarket, nutrition store, or neighborhood drugstore, there will usually be many types of fish oil available. As stated earlier, it is important to realize that all fish oils are not the same. The most common types that are available will say "Fish Oil 1,000 mg" on the label. It is important to note that for possible prevention or delay of Alzheimer's disease, patients need to take the right type of fish oil (capsules or liquid) and in adequate amounts. It is advised to look at the label and see the breakdown of how much DHA and EPA are in each serving, and how many capsules are needed for each serving size. Oftentimes, individuals will need to take at least two or three servings each day, or more, in order to get a suitable amount of these two omega-3 fatty acids. In general, I recommend that fish oil supplements must have DHA and EPA in them (the more DHA the better). Try to get at least 250 mg of DHA in each capsule for a total of at least 1,000–1,500 mg daily of DHA specifically. Fish oil should be started only under the supervision of a physician, and patients should try one capsule at first each day with a big meal and with water or juice, then increase if tolerated to one capsule twice per day after a week or so. It is suggested to start low and increase slowly, until an adequate total dose of DHA/EPA is achieved.

In the research studies that have been conducted, it seems that it may be necessary for patients to take even higher amounts of DHA than previously thought, such as 1,500–2,000 mg each day. The most recent data (published in November 2010 in *Alzheimer's and Dementia*, the journal of the Alzheimer's Association) showed that adults over the age of 55 with age-related cognitive decline demonstrated improvements in memory skills after taking 900 mg of algae-based DHA supplements each day (made by Martek). While there is much research that needs to be done to replicate these findings and clarify which types of fish oil work best, this evidence has led me to recommend fish oil supplements to patients at risk for AD. I base this on several studies. DHA supplementation, as was previously discussed in the Treatment section above, may more optimally slow cognitive decline in patients who are negative for the APOE4 gene. Further research is necessary to clarify this pharmacogenomic consideration.

When it comes to prevention, another study published several years ago (2006) showed that DHA 1,720 mg and EPA 600 mg each day showed benefits. In order to get this high amount of DHA, I tend to recommend a brand called Carlson Super DHA Gems, which have 500 mg of DHA per capsule. Another brand is Life's DHA (made by Martek and derived from algae, as discussed above), but any brand with a high amount of DHA (and some EPA) is suggested. Fish oil capsules usually have a varying amount (e.g., 1,000 mg) of *total* fish oil in each capsule, but each has a different amount of actual DHA/EPA. As an alternative to capsules, a liquid fish oil may be used. One brand to consider is called Nutri Supreme (available online at www.nutri-supreme.com or by calling 1-888-68-NUTRI), which is also kosher.

The cost of these supplements will depend on a

variety of factors. The price most significantly depends on the brand or strength of the fish oil and the location purchased. There is often a price difference between pharmacies in the same town and on Internet websites. It is advisable to shop around and visit several pharmacies, health food stores, and websites, and discuss with other caregivers, a social worker, or staff at the treating physician's office. It is imperative to pay close attention to the exact brand name, strength of each capsule, and serving size. The average cost of Carlson Super DHA Gems ranges from $30–$35 for 180 capsules, or $20–$25 per month (1,500 mg total DHA per day, 500 mg capsules), and the average cost of Life's DHA by Martek ranges from $22–$30 for 90 capsules, or $25 per month (900 mg total DHA per day, 300 mg capsules). As one example, the average cost for a 12-oz bottle of the Nutri-Supreme "Omega-3 GOLD" liquid fish oil (also contains 1,000 I.U. of vitamin D3 per teaspoon) is $43, or roughly $35 per month via the manufacturer's website.

Fish oil is generally safe but must be used under the supervision of a physician as there could be interactions with other medications the patient is taking. Fish oil may have an effect on bleeding and must be used with caution in patients on anticoagulant (blood thinner) medications like Coumadin (must have blood work monitored by a physician on a regular basis). Overall, fish oil is generally safe and also may have a beneficial effect on cholesterol, so I utilize this strategy frequently in my practice.

The other supplement that I often suggest is curcumin, also called turmeric root, which is the active ingredient in curry. There is no clear standardized dosing, and it is not currently known what dose or type is most beneficial. There are ongoing scientific trials that are studying this treatment, but since it is generally safe and there is some data to suggest its usefulness, I do recommend it in my clinical practice.

Curcumin can usually be purchased in a health food store and the directions on the bottle should always be followed. Since supplements are not regulated by the FDA and all brands are different in terms of dosage/strength, it is unclear which is best. In terms of safety, it is essential to make sure to discuss taking this supplement with the treating physician as there may be some potential for interactions with prescribed medications. The cost of curcumin varies widely depending on vendor, dosage, and strength, on average $10–$15 per month.

Vitamins

While there is no direct or clear scientific evidence (e.g., randomized, double-blinded placebo-controlled trials) that using vitamins will prevent or delay the onset of Alzheimer's disease, these interventions have a favorable risk-benefit ratio. In addition, some of these vitamins have scientific evidence that suggests there may be some benefit. I advocate for taking a multivitamin at least several times each week, and I also have patients consider taking folic acid (1 mg total per day), B_{12}, and vitamin D (1,000–2,000 I.U. per day, or more). As with all considerations, any supplement or vitamin must be taken with the approval and supervision of the treating physician (e.g., blood tests may need to be monitored), and further scientific studies are necessary in this area.

A recent study by de Jager and colleagues (*International Journal of Geriatric Psychiatry*, 2011) studied the effect of B vitamins on cognitive functioning and clinical decline. B vitamins are known to lower a biomarker in the blood called homocysteine, which has also been found to be a potential a risk factor for AD. In this double-blind study, MCI patients (ages 70 and above) with high homocysteine levels who received 0.8 mg of folic acid, 0.5 mg of vitamin B_{12} and 20 mg of vitamin B_6 each day has improved cognitive test scores on a variety of commonly performed tests. These included the Mini Mental State Examination (scored on a 0 to 30 point scale) and a "category fluency" test (e.g., how many different animals the patient can name in one minute). In this small study, B vitamins appeared to slow cognitive and clinical decline in people with MCI, in particular in those individuals with elevated homocysteine. Further studies are warranted to determine whether these vitamins may slow or prevent the progression from MCI to AD.

25. Can physical exercise help prevent Alzheimer's disease?

Yes! The importance of exercise, both physical and mental, cannot be stressed enough. The benefits of physical exercise in delaying the onset of Alzheimer's disease have been suggested in a variety of studies. As discussed earlier, levels of amyloid (the pathologic protein in the brain of Alzheimer's patients) occur many years before the onset of symptoms. There is research in lab animals (mice) that supports the use of exercise in order to decrease amyloid levels in the brain. In one study, mice that had Alzheimer's disease were put in two separate environments. Half the mice were very active and did physical exercise on a regular basis. The other mice did not have much physical activity at all. When they looked at the brains of the mice that exercised, the level of the "bad" Alzheimer's protein (amyloid) was cut in half! Studies in humans have also shown the cognitive benefits of exercise. Again, since we know that the accumulation of amyloid begins many years before the onset of symptoms, it is imperative that an active exercise regimen be incorporated into one's lifestyle as early as possible.

Considering this and based on my clinical experience, I am a strong advocate for increasing physical activity as tolerated and as approved by the patient's primary care physician. Oftentimes, I suggest a personal trainer if motivation is a problem, as physical exercise improves brain function as well as benefiting the rest of the body. I suggest exercise at least 3–4 times a week, for 45–60 minutes if tolerated. However, it is important to work up slowly to this regimen. As an example, if a patient does not get any exercise at all, even starting with a five minute walk once or twice a day is better than nothing. Ten minutes is better than five, twenty is better than ten, and so on. Some studies suggest that aerobic exercise is important, and other studies suggest that adding muscle mass through weight training is also helpful. We do not have enough scientific evidence to be able to tell which is better or in what combination, so I usually recommend a mixture of both, increasing as tolerated to the time periods listed above. When patients have mobility issues due to arthritis and other problems, pool therapy is an option to consider. Tai chi has also been studied and is an option. A home exercise program is also worthwhile to consider (e.g., workout DVDs, Nintendo Wii Fit Plus, and a variety of games on Microsoft Kinect).

26. Can mental exercise and cognitive activities help prevent Alzheimer's disease?

Increasing mental activity may also be helpful. Some suggestions that I recommend include video games like Brain Age, Big Brain Academy etc. (Nintendo DS or Nintendo Wii), puzzles, word games, reading books, crosswords, and other games requiring thought. Some studies suggest that the more one challenges the brain, the more one will be able to maintain it later (cognitive reserve hypothesis).

There are several resources that may be helpful, including brain teaser books. A good website mentioned earlier for brain activities that tracks patient progress is www.lumosity.com. Taking classes and learning a new language or a new skill may also be especially important. New hobbies and group socialization activities are also worthwhile.

The technique of "guided autobiography" is

currently being studied. This area was initially studied by Dr. James Birren as a method for helping individuals document their life stories in writing. There are a variety of live and online classes to learn more about this topic. In the future we hope to discover if this technique could be an effective means of delaying memory/cognitive decline.

In terms of cognitive exercise, I believe that the key is focusing on cognitive activities involving higher-order reasoning. What types of brain training works best? I do not typically recommend activities like sudoku, although I also do not discourage patients who enjoy it. I would rather that patients focus on more complicated cognitive tasks such as determining a "gist" message from a presentation, reading passage, or community lecture. Dr. Chapman and colleagues (2002) found that an individual's flexible ability to synthesize abstract meanings from details may help them to process information and remember those details. Gist reasoning training is where researchers train people to engage in abstract reasoning. As opposed to doing an activity such as sudoku (where repeated puzzles will only help to improve one's abilities at sudoku), gist reasoning activities will not only improve that activity, but there will also be a "spill over" effect. This means that other cognitive domains may improve aside from gist reasoning (Anand, Chapman, and colleagues, 2010).

27. Can music therapy and listening to music prevent Alzheimer's disease?

Listening to music (especially classical) and music therapy programs have been shown to improve memory in patients with Alzheimer's disease. Kraus and colleagues at Northwestern University (my brother's Alma Mater, Go Wildcats!) recently published exciting research showing that lifelong musical experiences can slow down brain aging and memory loss (*Neurobiology of Aging*, 2012). Music is a safe and enjoyable means of stimulating the mind and exercising memory, and may be recommended as part of an AD prevention plan. In fact, coupled with research by Merzenich and colleagues at the University of California–San Francisco, intensive musical training even late in life may improve brain function.

There is a helpful website that I tend to suggest for my patients called www.TherapyForMemory .com. There are several activities found on this website that may be beneficial. A recent study in the journal *Science* showed that listening to specific sounds while asleep led listeners to remember the sounds after they awoke. This is a very interesting finding and warrants further study. Going to a musical performance, the theater, or the symphony on a regular basis may be helpful. Learning how to play or even practicing an instrument that one has played in the past may also be worthwhile. I also suggest listening to music in the background (most of the evidence is for classical, but any enjoyable music could also work), as this may stimulate the mind passively and also help to improve learning and memory.

28. What types of nutritional or dietary changes may delay the onset of Alzheimer's disease?

There have been significant increases in the understanding of how diet and nutrition relate to the development of Alzheimer's disease. There are several specific dietary modifications that may delay the onset and/or progression of AD. Having a healthy diet that incorporates the points mentioned below is extremely important. Before making any dietary changes, they should of course be discussed with the patient's primary care physician or a dietician. Patients should be encouraged to utilize the combination of a balanced diet and good physical health, as they can work together to optimize health many years before the onset of Alzheimer's disease. In addition, it is important to mention some of the "practical" aspects of diet modification in an effort to delay the onset of AD. For myself, I have tried to make an honest effort over the last several years to follow many of the suggestions that I advocate. There are some days and weeks where I am quite disciplined, and others where I am much less adherent. It is important to not let frustration get the best of you and to realize that even subtle dietary changes for a few days per week, or a few weeks per month, may lead to long-term benefits when followed for many years in a row.

In the back of the book in the Resources section, there are several examples of food choices to consider and which may be better for optimal brain health. There is also a section on food terminology, to help you understand dietary choices that present themselves throughout the day. These two sections were added to this edition based on feedback from readers like you. In fact, we received so much positive feedback about the diet and nutrition sections in this book that we are now working a new book focusing solely on diet and nutrition for AD. You can visit www.TheADdiet.com for more information, or to complete a reader survey about this book, please visit www.TheADplan.com/Survey. Your input and time are both greatly appreciated!

There is still much research that needs to be

done about dietary interventions for prevention of AD. This research is unfortunately difficult to perform and is rigorous due to the long length of the studies and the many variables that come into play. In June 2011, Craft and colleagues published a fascinating paper (*Archives of Neurology*) supporting that "consumption of a diet high in saturated fat and simple carbohydrates may contribute to pathologic processes in the brain that increase the risk of Alzheimer's disease, while a diet low in saturated fat and simple carbohydrates may offer protection against dementia and enhance brain health." In the coming years I am hopeful that we will learn a great deal more about this area, but in the meantime, further scientific research on diet and nutrition in AD is warranted.

Let's review nutritional aspects that should not be overlooked when attempting to delay the onset of Alzheimer's. Before we discuss which specific types of food and beverage choices are best, it is important to first obtain a basic understanding of the fundamentals of AD nutrition, as it will help patients and caregivers make the right food choices. Much of the following text is repeated from Section 2, as the same basic concepts apply. However, in this section, I have given a few "real-life" examples of my personal decisions regarding food choices that may reduce my risk of developing AD.

As mentioned earlier, last year I spoke with a nutritional scientist who also has a strong family history of Alzheimer's disease. I asked him the following question: What is the number-one thing that you would suggest to potentially delay the onset of Alzheimer's? His response was simple—a low-carbohydrate diet, avoiding simple sugars. Now let's discuss what he meant by simple sugars, and then review the reasons why such diet modifications may be important.

There are three different types of "macro" nutrients, which most people are familiar with. These are proteins, fats, and carbohydrates. Some examples of protein sources that I recommend include fish high in DHA (e.g., wild salmon, mackerel, lake trout, herring, sardines, albacore tuna), poultry (skinless chicken and turkey), and lean meats (beef), which are hormone free when possible, egg whites, and low-fat (or non-fat) dairy products. Monosaturated fats (e.g., extra-virgin olive oil, peanuts, avocados) and polyunsaturated fats (e.g., nuts and seeds) in moderation are advisable. Avoiding trans fats and saturated fats is of very high importance. I also suggest minimizing "simple sugars." Examples of simple sugars include the type of sugar that is put into coffee (cane sugar), as well as more concentrated versions such as high fructose corn syrup and corn syrup in general.

There are two different types of sugars: "added sugars" and "naturally occurring" sugars. An added sugar is a sugar or syrup that is added to foods during processing or preparation. These do not include naturally occurring sugars such as fructose (in fruits) or lactose (in milk products). All sugars/carbohydrates, regardless of whether they are added or naturally occurring, can be characterized in terms of their glycemic index.

The term "glycemic index" is important to understand. Just like the different types of fish oil described above, all carbohydrates are not created equal. Glycemic index refers to a classification proposed to quantify the relative blood glucose response to carbohydrate-containing foods (cited from www.health.gov). In other words, for any carbohydrate that is eaten (e.g., cane sugar vs. pasta), the glycemic index describes how much insulin is released by the body in response.

There are several theories that hypothesize why minimizing carbohydrates may be useful. One theory relates to the production of ketone bodies, which can be used as an alternative fuel source for the brain and may help reduce oxidative damage inside the brain cells (mitochondria). This is covered in greater detail in Chapter 8.

Another theory is based on the role of insulin, especially as it relates to consumption of high glycemic index carbohydrates. Insulin's effects on aging of the brain have been studied in detail. Regulating insulin "signaling" affects longevity and has a role in normal and pathological brain aging (Barbieri, 2003). Insulin receptors are densely packed in the hippocampus (the memory center in the brain), and insulin itself has a direct influence on the brain since it enters via crossing into the blood-brain barrier (Apelt, 2001). Insulin also modulates neurotransmitters in the brain and is involved with memory.

Insulin resistance is a condition where insulin cannot carry out its usual activities. Insulin resistance is associated with a variety of medical conditions, including obesity, diabetes, high blood pressure, and high cholesterol (among others).

In addition, insulin and beta-amyloid are related. Studies have shown that insulin raises beta-amyloid (the pathologic protein found in the brain of patients with Alzheimer's disease) in older adults (over 70 years old) and also increases inflammation in the brain (Watson, 2003).

Now that we have discussed the importance of insulin, you can better understand why minimizing simple carbohydrates is a sensible idea. Simple carbohydrates are composed of a single sugar molecule or two joined sugar molecules, such as glucose, fructose, lactose, and sucrose. Simple carbohydrates include white and brown sugar, fruit sugar, corn syrup, molasses, honey, and candy. Avoiding this type of sugar completely is very difficult, if not impossible. However, with dedication and education, many of my patients have made constructive changes to their diets.

Overall, reducing "added sugars" and selecting complex carbohydrates (as opposed to simple carbohydrates) as part of a balanced diet is most important. Complex carbohydrates are defined as large chains of sugar units arranged to form starches and fiber. These include vegetables, whole fruits, grains (brown rice, buckwheat, quinoa, oats, wheat, barley, corn), and legumes (chick peas, black-eyed peas, lentils, as well as beans such as lima, kidney, pinto, soy, and black beans). Starchy foods like pasta and white rice break down quickly to sugar and thus should be minimized.

When educating my patients, I again pass on the advice of a great scholar who taught me several things prior to medical school—my mother. "Everything in moderation" is what she emphasized. When making changes to one's diet, old habits are hard to break. In my clinical practice, I am more insistent on these types of dietary modifications to be made slowly but surely even beginning in patients many decades before the possible onset of symptoms of AD. Several children, and siblings, of patients with AD have scheduled appointments to see me for "Alzheimer's prevention," and no matter if they are in their 30s, 40s, 50s, 60s, or beyond, I advocate strongly for attention to diet and nutrition.

A recent study by Dr. Craft and colleagues compared two different types of dietary interventions on cognitive outcomes: A Western-style diet (consisting of high saturated fat and high sugar) vs. a Mediterranean-style diet (consisting of low saturated fat and low glycemic index carbohydrates). See Chapter 10 for more information on this study. Another recent study published by Krikorian and colleagues compared a high-carbohydrate diet vs. a very low-carbohydrate diet in patients with mild cognitive impairment (*Neurobiology of Aging*, 2010). This was a randomized study of 23 patients over 6 weeks. This study showed significant benefits in the low-carbohydrate group in verbal memory, in addition to weight loss, decreased waist circumference, decreased fasting blood sugar, and decreased fasting insulin. While further studies are warranted to determine preventative potential and to investigate the biological reasons why these diet changes may work, this is exciting evidence that has reinforced the dietary suggestions I make to my patients at risk.

When individuals follow a very low-carbohydrate diet, this will lead to a state of brain/body metabolism called "ketosis." However, following this type of very low-carbohydrate diet is very difficult, and most are unable to adhere. As a compromise, I will occasionally advocate for the "early-bird" special technique when it comes to dietary modification. While I am from New York, I have been living in Miami for several years, and my entire immediate family moved to South Florida in 1997. Soon after the move, I learned that an "early-bird" special was a technique offering special pricing deals when eating dinner before 6 pm at several restaurants. Not only can you save some money, but there may also be a brain-boosting effect of this strategy! In some patients, and only when approved by their primary care physician, waiting at least 12 hours in between dinner and breakfast can bring about a very mild state of "ketosis." This technique, combined with minimal (if any) carbohydrates in the morning, requires further research, but may make sense from this brain/body metabolism perspective. There is some scientific evidence that a state of ketosis may have "anti-aging" effects on the brain. As such, even trying this approach several days a week may be a reasonable option to reduce risk. Of course, this means no late-night snacking between dinner and breakfast.

Personally, and due to a variety of reasons, several times per week I end up skipping breakfast. On a typical evening, I will finish dinner by 7 pm, and my next meal may not be until noon the following day. While this mild state of ketosis may be protective for me, I am unsure of the exact benefit. Regardless, it is a strategy that fits with my lifestyle, work habits, and schedule, and has been approved by my own primary care physician. The scientific data on "skipping breakfast" is mixed, but what is clear is that it may depend on the person. While controversial, this strategy works for me, leads to my consuming fewer overall calories during the day, and also fits with my personal preference of morning exercise (as exercise may have a greater benefit after a night of fasting, in that a person will burn most calories from fat instead of carbohydrates).

I try to minimize carbohydrates when possible, especially added sugar. Any time I take a drink of juice, I will "water it down" by more than half, plus ice. My one weakness is too much dark chocolate; however, I have been able to cut this down significantly over the last several years. I always choose lean meats when possible, and for the most part, I avoid fried and fatty foods. I drink only skim milk, and choose non-fat or low-fat dairy options when possible. I drink coffee in moderation, eat green leafy vegetables and fruits as often as I can, and fish at least twice per week.

Now, reducing carbohydrates in the diet is easier said than done! As an example, on the way to the airport recently, I ran into some traffic and as such didn't have time to grab dinner before boarding my flight. It was 9 pm, I was hungry, and my food choices were limited. After takeoff I asked the flight attendant about the snack options, and she replied "we have a jumbo-sized cookie, potato chips, or cheese and crackers." Starving, and justifying my expenditure on "market research" purposes for this chapter, I decided to buy all three.

Before deciding which of these would be my dinner for the evening, I read the nutrition facts label, as I have become accustomed to over the last several years. Let's start with the cookie: 150 calories; total fat 6 grams (3 g saturated, 0 g trans fat); cholesterol 5 mg; sodium 115 mg; carbohydrates

23 g (dietary fiber 0 g, sugars 13 g); protein 2 g. At first glance, the cookie was not as "bad" for me as I had expected. I then did a double take at the label and noticed the serving size of each cookie is three, meaning I needed to triple the amounts above if I would have eaten the whole thing. At that point I decide to gift the cookie to the passenger in the seat next to me (who proceeded to eat it quickly, and then fall asleep drooling, within minutes of finishing it entirely).

With my options for dinner dwindling by the minute, I reviewed the next option on the menu: the cheese and crackers. This plastic-wrapped tray consisted of four butter crackers (.5 oz, but no nutrition facts on the label), one piece of pasteurized processed cheddar cheese (.75 oz, also no nutrition facts on the label), a box of raisins (1 oz, 90 calories, 0 g fat, 5 mg sodium; total carbohydrates 22 g [dietary fiber 2 g, sugars 20 g]; protein 1 g); and a bag of mixed nuts (170 calories, 15 g fat (2 g saturated, 0 g trans fat); cholesterol 0 g; sodium 110 mg; total carbohydrates 6 g [dietary fiber 2 g, sugars 1 g]; protein 5 g).

Now, upon review of this smorgasbord of packaged options, we run into several key considerations that make healthy eating somewhat more of a challenge. Most important, several items in this package come without any documented evidence of the dietary value of their components. With some education and experience, one can certainly "guesstimate" the contents, but knowing for sure will always be a challenge.

The third and final option is the potato chips. This time I noticed the "fine print" staring at me right at the top of the nutrition facts label. In this 6-oz container, we have 6 servings (1 oz each) with each serving consisting of 150 calories; total fat 9 grams (1.5 g saturated, 0 g trans fat, 3.5 g polyunsaturated, 2.5 g monounsaturated); cholesterol 0 mg; sodium 140 mg; carbohydrates 16 g (dietary fiber 1g, sugars 1 g); protein 1g.

Alas, when I began to do the math here, I realized that the options presented to me were less than optimal. Having a family history of AD, being a practicing physician, and being an advocate for diet modification to both reduce the risk for and improve the management of AD, I try to make healthy food choices whenever possible. When I was younger, I would have started with the cookie, then continued with half (~3 oz or so) of the potato chips, and maybe finished with my "dessert" of one piece of cheese and a few of the butter crackers. On this evening, however, I went with the bag of nuts, and the box of raisins, before realizing that I had saved a "protein bar" in my laptop bag just in case of an event like this. For my beverage selection, I first had a full glass of water, and then a half a glass of cranberry juice and ice, mixed with water (as I mentioned before, another easy way to cut down the carbs, in half).

Related to dietary changes, it is essential to avoid being overweight. Patients who want to lower their risk of developing AD should be encouraged to lose weight through a structured intervention program incorporating both diet and exercise. This program must be supervised by the treating physician.

How is obesity related to cognition? Increased body-mass index (BMI) and increased waist-to-hip ratio is linked to hippocampal volume in later life. Also, having high central adiposity (also known as a big "gut" or stomach) increases the risk of cognitive impairment (Whitmer and Yaffe, *Neurology*, 2008).

Metabolic syndrome has also been linked to increased cognitive aging and is defined as a constellation of vascular risk factors including increased waist circumference, low HDL cholesterol, high triglycerides, high blood pressure, and high fasting blood glucose.

In summary, obesity and metabolic syndrome are both associated with accelerated cognitive aging, especially in individuals with medical illnesses that cause inflammation in the body.

Considering the information presented above, some believe that adopting a Mediterranean-style diet may be helpful toward delaying the onset of AD. Fruits and vegetables, lean protein (fish, chicken, turkey), low-fat foods (especially low in saturated fats), nuts, and seeds are a part of this type of diet. Some advocate for minimizing consumption of red meat (no more than 1–2 times per week) and also minimizing the amount of processed foods in the diet.

When it comes to dietary choices, here are two good rules of thumb:

1. The fewer ingredients listed on the nutrition

label—the better! (Suggestion courtesy of Cheryl Fawn.)

2. When eating dairy products, consider low-fat (or better yet, non-fat) options when possible.

We have talked about the importance of "good fat" or unsaturated fat, vs. "bad fat," or saturated and trans fats. It is important to learn the difference and make a habit of reading nutrition labels. In fact, it is important to read the "Nutrition Facts" information and ingredient list on foods when available. Reading labels will help keep track of exactly what is put into the body, which in turn has an effect on brain health.

While taking supplements, capsules, liquids, etc. that contain omega-3 fatty acids, higher amounts of DHA than EPA is most important. Eating fish that are high in DHA/EPA is also advisable. There are several specific types of fish, including mackerel, lake trout, herring, sardines, albacore tuna, and wild salmon that are high in these two kinds of omega-3 fatty acids. Tofu and other forms of soybeans may be helpful, as well as canola, walnut, and their oils. I advocate for patients to eat fish in moderation, roughly twice a week, to ensure a good supply of DHA and EPA while mitigating the potential for increasing mercury in the diet. The types of fish that are chosen are also important (e.g., if the fish is farm-raised rather than wild-caught, the level of omega-3s may be significantly less).

Antioxidants in the diet are also very important. There are ongoing studies to determine whether eating a diet rich in antioxidants is helpful for cognition. Considering the risk-benefit ratio I recommend incorporating antioxidant-rich foods into the diet. One study is looking at the combination of omega-3 fatty acids plus blueberry powder. The investigators will be capturing data on metabolic parameters, inflammation, and uptake of omega-3 fatty acids, as well as the effects on cognition.

There are several antioxidant-rich foods aside from blueberries that I recommend, and these include several types of berries (e.g., raspberries, cranberries, acai, cherries, strawberries, blackberries, and elderberries). Other fruits like tomatoes (try heating them as this may increase the availability of the antioxidants to the body), pomegranates, red grapes (and grape juice), oranges, grapefruits, and apples are also high in antioxidants. I suggest at least 1–2 servings per day.

There are a variety of vegetables that are high in substances that may protect the brain. These include carrots, broccoli, beets, spinach, kale, cabbage, Brussels sprouts, artichokes, collard, and other dark leafy greens. Other high antioxidant foods include walnuts, pecans, dark chocolate, teas (green and black), and coffee (we will cover this in greater detail later).

Another recent study in animals looked at the combination of a diet high in antioxidants together with behavioral enrichment. Researchers have studied these interventions in dogs (beagles) since older animals develop a syndrome that is similar to Alzheimer's disease in humans. Dogs that develop cognitive deficits in middle age may be diagnosed with something commonly known as "doggie Alzheimer's" or the more official term, canine cognitive dysfunction syndrome. These dogs give scientists a model that is similar to Alzheimer's (but not exactly the same). You can read more about this study in the introduction to Section 3, or in Chapter 10. The take-home point of this research is that the combined intervention of an antioxidant-rich diet plus exercise led to improved mitochondrial function and better enabled protective mechanisms in the brain of the dogs. While these studies need to be replicated in humans, it seems that exercise and behavioral enrichment synergize with diet to enhance brain health.

As such I advocate for these changes to be made by my patients who want to lower their risk of AD. I also suggest integrating socialization elements into exercise. These "social" aspects may prove to be an important aspect toward maximizing brain health. Again, translating these findings to humans is necessary and will take several years, but why wait? Considering the risk-benefit ratio, this is a strategy that should be considered.

While some clinicians advocate for taking vitamins in pill form, a balanced diet should provide most of the daily vitamin requirements. Ensuring adequate intake of vitamins such as folic acid, B_6 and B_{12} are important, as is vitamin D (see pages 173–174 for more details). Several studies have shown that a significant proportion of people are deficient in vitamin D, and that supplementation may be beneficial for brain protection. As such, I have recently started to consider adding 1,000–2,000 I.U. (or more) of vitamin D in pill form, along with at least 10–15 minutes of sunlight per day. The exact dose of vitamin D is unclear at this time. Due to this uncertainty (e.g., dose, whether or not a blood level should be drawn), the decision to take vitamins and in what amounts should always be discussed with and approved by the patient's primary care physician.

There has been a lot of talk in the media about whether caffeine and coffee should be considered in the treatment plan of AD. Caffeine may have effects on the heart (such as increasing heart rate) and may increase anxiety. However, several studies (mostly in Europe) have shown the potential for a "protective" effect of caffeine/coffee on the brain. More research needs to be done in this area; however, the most recent study in mice yielded some very interesting results. Cao and colleagues found that mice with Alzheimer's that drank the human equivalent of several cups of coffee each day had cognitive benefits (*Journal of Alzheimer's Disease*, 2011). While there are no scientific studies in humans that clearly address this, I again use my mom's rule of "everything in moderation." A few cups, or perhaps several, earlier in the day are probably okay, as long as this has been approved by the treating physician.

The effect of alcohol consumption on AD prevention is currently unclear. One serving (in women) or one to two servings (in men) per day may be reasonable. A recent article by Neafsey and Collins concluded that this amount may reduce the risk of dementia and cognitive decline (*Neuropsychiatric Disease and Treatment*, 2011) although further studies are warranted. I advise against consumption of more than two servings per day in my patients, as this may lead to significant health consequences.

To summarize, I suggest focusing on these general categories of diet and nutrition. When making such dietary changes, it may be helpful to keep a diet journal (www.TheADplan.com) and keep a meal log in order to keep track of what is eaten. It is also advisable to have laboratory studies (blood work) done before making changes to the diet, as well as several weeks or months afterwards. Again, any and all changes should be under the guidance and strict supervision of a physician and dietician.

TOP TEN DIET AND NUTRITION RECOMMENDATIONS

1. Include the following suggested breakdown of macronutrients (modified from Craft study):

   • Fat: 25% (<7% of which saturated)

   • Carbohydrates: 30–45% (low glycemic index)

   • Protein: 25–35%

2. Minimize carbohydrates with a high glycemic index—especially added simple sugars, high fructose corn syrup, and corn syrup in general.

   It is unclear what the exact target number of total carbs should be per day, but some suggest 130 grams/day (low-carb diet). Others suggest significantly less, even less than half that amount, for a very low-carbohydrate (ketogenic) diet. Decrease dietary carbs slowly over weeks and with supervision and approval by a physician (see sample plan below). Some experts feel that to have more of a significant benefit from decreasing carbohydrate intake, a very low-carb diet is necessary. While I do not wholeheartedly disagree with this, the difficulty with which a very low-carb diet presents itself has fostered me to take a much more moderate approach with this strategy. I therefore do not yet widely recommend this method; however, further study is warranted in the future. Patients with health conditions (e.g., diabetes) should avoid ketogenic diets as severe health consequences may occur.

3. Try a Mediterranean-style diet, including fruits and vegetables, lean protein (fish, chicken, turkey), low-fat items, nuts, and seeds. Avoid excessive red meat intake as well as processed foods.

4. "Good" fat (unsaturated) vs. "bad" fat (saturated and trans fats)—learn the difference and avoid the "bad" fats!

5. Omega-3 fatty acids (DHA and EPA).

6. Antioxidants.

7. Vitamins—folic acid, B_6, B_{12}, vitamin D (via adequate nutrition, or supplement as needed in pill or liquid form).

8. In general, the fewer ingredients listed on the label, the better!

9. Low-fat dairy products (or non-fat) when possible.

10. Coffee (caffeinated): a few or perhaps several cups earlier in the day may be beneficial.

Regarding recommendation #2, when making dietary suggestions for my patients, I suggest the following step-wise approach toward dietary enhancement. Since there are potential negative health consequences of the diet plan below (as a patient's medical history needs to be considered before making such recommendations), any and all changes in diet need to be supervised and approved by the treating physician. For example, patients with diabetes who are predisposed to a condition called ketoacidosis should not follow the diet below. Other potential side effects that have been reported from low-carbohydrate diets include constipation or diarrhea, headaches, and muscle weakness.

Week 1

DO NOT make any drastic changes to the diet. During the first week patients should become more "mindful" of what they are eating, look closer at nutrition labels and ingredients, and go food shopping at a variety of grocery and health food stores. This should help with education regarding what types of foods may be most favorable to eat. Read and re-read the recommendations above and below several times, and compare the food choices that have been made in the past with the choices planned for the future. Buy a scale (with body fat analyzer) and begin a weekly log of weight, percent body fat, waist circumference, and activity level (include number of exercise sessions per week and total amount of exercise time). Record this information on diet journal log sheets found at www.TheADplan.com, and include all meals for two days during the week (e.g., Wednesday and Saturday).

Week 2

Continue diet log sheets as instructed above, and keep track of total grams of carbohydrates as best as possible. A variety of websites and handbooks can give estimates. Once approved by and only under close supervision of a physician, try for a goal of

130–150 grams of carbohydrates per day, and minimize those with a high glycemic index. Begin efforts to follow the general breakdown of macronutrients per day as described above (protein vs. fat vs. carbohydrates) and increase lean meats and low-fat options, while decreasing simple and added sugars. Try to eat fish at least twice this week, increase fruits, vegetables, and other foods rich in antioxidants.

Weeks 3–4

Continue diet log sheets as instructed above. Keep track of total grams of carbohydrates as best as possible, and try for a goal of 110–130 grams of carbohydrates per day. Minimize those carbohydrates with a high glycemic index. Follow the general breakdown of macronutrients per day above (protein vs. fat vs. carbohydrates). Continue a step-wise increase in lean meats and low fat options, while decreasing simple and added sugars. Try to eat fish at least two to three times each week, continue to increase foods rich in antioxidants, and increase fruits and vegetables.

Weeks 5–6

Continue as above but now try to decrease carbohydrates to 90–110 grams per day. Minimize carbs with a high glycemic index.

Weeks 7–8

Continue as above but now try to decrease carbohydrates to 70–90 grams per day. Minimize those with a high glycemic index. If any symptoms of ketoacidosis occur (Early signs: increasing fatigue, tired and sleepy, weakness, increased thirst, frequent urination, dry skin and tongue, leg cramps, fruity odor to the breath, upset stomach, nausea. Later signs: vomiting, shortness of breath, increased breathing rate or pulse), increase the amount of carbohydrates in the diet, and speak with the primary care doctor or treating physician immediately. If symptoms are moderate or severe, go to the emergency room or see the primary care doctor or supervising physician immediately.

Week 9 and beyond

Continue diet as tolerated. Decrease carbs to 65 grams or less per day if tolerated. If symptoms of ketoacidosis occur (Early signs: increasing fatigue, tired and sleepy, weakness, increased thirst, frequent urination, dry skin and tongue, leg cramps, fruity odor to the breath, upset stomach, nausea. Later signs: vomiting, shortness of breath, increased breathing rate or pulse), increase the amount of carbohydrates, and speak with the primary care doctor/treating physician. If symptoms are moderate or severe, go to the emergency room or see a primary care or supervising physician immediately.

~

While it may be necessary to have even less carbs than the amounts detailed above, any attempt at a very low-carbohydrate (ketogenic) diet must be made under the close supervision of a treating physician. Diabetics should avoid ketogenic diets, as severe health consequences may occur.

29. What other life interventions, like stress modification or increasing social interactions, may have an impact on preventing AD?

Ongoing follow-up with the one's primary care physician is imperative for routine health maintenance. Any vascular risk factors (high blood pressure, cholesterol, diabetes/high sugars, etc.) have the potential to increase progression of memory decline and may cause AD to occur sooner than it otherwise would have. Patients should have cholesterol results checked and consider treatment. While unproven, cholesterol drugs, also known as statin medications, may provide benefits and slow cognitive decline. Further studies are warranted to address this and the risks and benefits of statin use should be discussed in detail with the treating physician. In those patients who are at risk, I tend to suggest statin therapy in patients with borderline or high cholesterol. I will even on occasion consider using these medications in low doses in patients with near normal cholesterol, in case they could potentially prevent or slow disease progression. This is a complex decision that must be balanced with the risk-benefit ratio of this type of therapy.

The potential for "neuroprotection" with therapies such as the medical food caprylic triglyceride (Axona) have yet to be determined. Inducing ketosis may help to protect mitochondria by reducing oxidative damage, but there are no data and no trials that have studied Axona in terms of prevention or delaying the onset of AD. When dogs are fed medium-chain triglycerides (like Axona), there is some evidence that shows increased mitochondrial efficiency and less oxidative damage. While this is an intriguing finding, the use of Axona off-label to delay onset of AD will continue to be controversial, until proven. In my practice, I have used this strategy in a few very select patients with mild cognitive impairment who desire "anything and everything" to be done, and who accept the associated risk-benefit ratio.

Additional strategies that are important include

managing everyday psychosocial stress (which has a cumulative negative effect over time), minimizing major traumatic stress, increasing social interactions, learning new skills, and getting involved in new hobbies.

Stress

Repetitive thought processes, or ruminating over negative thoughts, can take relatively minor stressors and transform them into more significant outcomes (Stawski and Rosnick, 2007).

Individuals who refrain from ruminating may respond differently to life stressors and may have improved outcomes on memory and thinking. In fact, it is not the stress itself, but the perception and processing of the stress that is the most important on which to focus.

Individuals who have repeated distress and have trouble dealing with that distress have been found to: (1) have worse cognitive health outcomes, and (2) have smaller brain volumes.

The term *neuroticism* reflects an individual's tendency to respond to a stressor with a disproportionate amount of negativity. Stress has been shown to increase rates of cognitive decline, and daily stress decreases working memory (even stress over a one-day time span). In fact, ongoing work and/or life stress over time can age the brain by up to four years! Individuals who respond more negatively to minor daily hassles may have increased memory and thinking impairment as they age.

Worry or rumination (unconstructive repetitive thoughts) causes decreased performance on cognitive testing (Brasschot, Thayer, and Gerin 2006). Worry also has independent negative cardiac effects.

What is it about neuroticism that causes this decline? Ongoing research is studying this question, and some hypotheses include effects on metabolic risk factors and sleep quality.

Markers of neuroticism, most significantly anxiety and vulnerability to stress, are associated with more rapid cognitive decline and higher likelihood of developing AD (Wilson, 2003). These negative effects of neuroticism, including psychological stress, occur many years before the onset of symptoms and are a direct risk factor for the disease.

The stress response, when prolonged over a

long period of time, leads to worse cognitive outcomes. Studies have shown that decreasing stress may actually have a positive effect on brain regions that are involved in memory (Holzel, Lazar and colleagues, 2008–2009). Some interventions that are considered to combat this "brain stress" include yoga, meditation, and self-esteem therapy, although additional studies need to be performed in order to confirm this.

Low self-esteem has also been shown to exacerbate the stress response. Psychosocial challenges combined with negative feedback may also influence stress-hormone release and may correlate with smaller volumes of the memory center of the brain (hippocampus).

Social Interactions

A variety of research has studied social interactions, including social ties and networking, and their effects on cognitive functioning. We are unsure of why or how more rigorous social relationships may protect memory. One thought is that hormonal factors may mediate stress and thus be protective.

The interactions between social, psychological, and physical activities are important, as they work in combination to maintain cognition and possibly protect from later decline. From an intervention perspective, multimodal programs that are integrated into everyday life will likely yield the most benefit.

The best advice I can give was shared with me by my friend Hector, a fellow Yankee fan and colleague who has dedicated himself tirelessly toward helping patients and caregivers with AD. His mother suffered from Alzheimer's, his father was her devoted caregiver, and I was fortunate to spend some time with him a few years ago helping to raise awareness of AD. He simply said, "Stay engaged in life!" These are the exact words I say virtually every day to those who are worried about developing AD.

30. Can you summarize the most optimal prevention plan for AD?

A combination of pharmacologic and non-pharmacologic interventions many years before the potential onset of Alzheimer's may delay the onset, or decrease the severity of, Alzheimer's and possibly other associated cognitive impairments (age-related cognitive decline, vascular dementia).

While it is our hope that these interventions will one day be proven to even possibly prevent the onset of AD, further well-designed scientific studies are certainly warranted. These studies will take many years and many hundreds of millions of dollars. In the meantime, I take the approach of considering the risk-benefit ratio when suggesting the following interventions for patients that I care for in my clinical practice.

Top Ten Considerations for Alzheimer's Prevention

1. **Increase physical activity** as tolerated and as approved by the primary care physician. Suggest personal trainer if motivation is a problem, as physical exercise improves brain function as well as benefiting the rest of the body. Recommend exercise at least 3–4 times a week, for 45–60 minutes if tolerated. If the patient is overweight, it is important to try to lose weight over time through a combination of diet and exercise.

2. **Maintain a healthy diet** (discuss with primary care physician or dietician). Follow the diet and nutrition guidelines listed in Chapter 28, incorporating a Mediterranean-style diet, including fruits and vegetables, lean protein (fish, chicken, turkey), low-fat items, nuts, and seeds. Avoid excessive red meat and processed foods.

Increase antioxidants. Most important, decrease carbohydrates, especially high glycemic carbs like simple sugars. Fish like mackerel, lake trout, herring, sardines, albacore tuna, and wild salmon are high in two kinds of omega-3 fatty acids: eicosapentaenoic acid (EPA) and docosahexaenoic acid (DHA).

3. **Increase socialization**, including activity programs, adult-education classes, and social groups. Learning a new language, studying a new subject, or taking up new hobbies, especially in group settings, may be especially useful.

4. **De-stress!** First identify and then reduce life stressors. Think positively and see the primary care physician (or psychiatrist) for general guidance. Consider a therapist if stress is a significant problem. Try to keep life in balance. Consider meditation, yoga, and other enjoyable relaxing/calming activities. Adequate sleep is also essential. Learn more about sleep hygiene and be sure to get a medical evaluation by the treating physician if there is difficulty sleeping or if extreme fatigue is felt during the day.

5. **Increase mental activity,** including video games like Brain Age, Big Brain Academy, etc. (Nintendo DS or Nintendo Wii). Puzzles, word games, reading books, crosswords, and other games requiring thought may also be helpful a few times per week (challenging the brain may help maintain it). There is a website called www.lumosity.com, which is a good resource for brain activities that tracks patient progress. I recommend using the program once per week.

6. **Listen to music** (especially classical) and consider music activity and educational programs that can be found on the website www.TherapyForMemory.com.

7. **Ongoing follow-up with the primary care doctor** for routine health maintenance. Any vascular risk factors (high blood pressure, cholesterol, diabetes/high sugars, etc.) will increase the rate of memory decline. Have cholesterol results checked and consider treatment (while unproven, cholesterol medications [statins] may provide benefits and slow cognitive decline.

Risks and benefits of statin use should be discussed in detail with the treating physician. If diagnosed with high blood pressure, consider treatment with an ACE inhibitor (e.g., lisinopril, perindopril, or captopril as they cross the blood-brain barrier). There may be some protective benefits of ACE inhibitors (research is ongoing, albeit unproven).

8. **Assure adequate dietary intake of essential vitamins.** Consider a multivitamin each day, folic acid 1 mg (total) each day, B_{12}, and vitamin D 1,000–2,000 I.U. each day (or perhaps more) may also be beneficial (further scientific studies are necessary). Risk-benefit ratio should be discussed in detail with treating physician (and certain blood tests may need to be monitored or performed). Consider about 10–15 minutes of sunlight per day.

9. **Curcumin** (turmeric root). Buy in a health food store.

10. **Fish oil supplements** (must have DHA and EPA in it; the more DHA, the better). Try to

get at least 250 mg of DHA in each capsule for a total of at least 1,000–1,500 mg daily of DHA specifically. At first try one capsule each day with a big meal (with water or juice), then increase if tolerated to one capsule twice per day after a week or so. It is suggested to start low and increase slowly, until an adequate total dose of DHA/EPA is achieved. Consider Carlson Super DHA Gems, which have 500 mg of DHA and 200 mg of EPA per capsule; another brand is Life's DHA (Martek), but any brand with a high amount of DHA may be suggested. (Fish oil capsules usually have 1,000 mg of TOTAL fish oil in each capsule, but each has a varied amount of actual DHA.) As an alternative, a liquid fish oil may be used (consider Nutri Supreme Omega-3 EPA/DHA, 888-68-NUTRI, www.nutri-supreme.com).

Conclusion

When I gave my first lecture on Alzheimer's disease in the early 2000s, my comments were limited to fifteen minutes on treatment and zero minutes on prevention. Today, I can spend up to an hour and a half on the topic of treatment, and over an hour on the topic prevention alone. In fact, just within the past year, and for the first time in my career, I was invited to speak on the topic of Alzheimer's prevention at conferences ranging from our local University of Miami Miller School of Medicine Department of Neurology annual Neuro-Update course, to the World Congress of the American Academy of Anti-Aging Medicine.

If this trend is any indication of the future landscape of AD, then we can feel reassured that science and medicine have the power to combat this most devastating disease. Additionally, the National Alzheimer's Project Act (NAPA) was recently signed into law. NAPA is an unprecedented effort that will help to create a coordinated national strategy to battle the most challenging public health crisis facing our nation today. In 2011, baby boomers began to turn 65. Considering that the number-one risk factor for AD is advancing age, the importance of NAPA cannot be overstated.

NAPA will help lead our government to create a national strategic plan to overcome the AD epidemic across the spectrum of patient care, research, and caregiver support. An emphasis will be placed on institutional, home- and community-based programs and their outcomes. In February 2012, the President announced plans to spend an additional $156 million dollars for research and caregiver support. Patients and caregivers may derive solace in the fact that our government is slowly but surely stepping up efforts against AD, a disease that is bound to touch all of us.

I remain steadfast in my commitment and look forward to the next decade of advances in Alzheimer's treatment and prevention.

Reader Survey

If after reading this book, you would like to share your comments and suggestions on how to make future editions more helpful for you, please visit this link to complete a brief reader survey and enter code FREE2013:

www.TheADplan.com/Survey

Prior to release of the 2013 edition, we will randomly select 50 people who completed the survey and send out a free copy of the book when it is released. In addition, and as a special token of our thanks, we will enter you in a raffle for a $100 Amazon giftcard. Several suggestions were incorporated into this edition thanks to readers just like you, and we value your input. Also, to join our free e-mail newsletter, visit:

www.TheADplan.com/Newsletter.php

RESOURCES

APPENDIX A.
Helpful Websites Cited in This Book

www.TheADplan.com
Visit for Updates to this Book, Latest AD
News/Blog, AD Diet Journal Log Sheets,
Reader Reviews, and much more

www.TherapyForMemory.com
Latest Information on How to Fight Memory
Loss, Ask the Experts Section, and Doctor-
Recommended Brain Stimulating Activities
(like the inexpensive Music Activity and
Educational Program and Soothing Music
to listen to while sleeping)

www.TheADdiet.com
Coming Soon! Detailed Diet Plan
for Treatment/Prevention

www.lumosity.com
Brain Activity Program to Use Weekly
and Track Progress

www.alz.org
Caregiver Resources, Support Groups
and Information and Educational
Opportunities about AD

www.alzfdn.org
Information and Resources about AD
for Patients/Families

www.health.gov
Helpful Educational Information
about Health and Nutrition

www.nia.nih.gov/alzheimers
Excellent Overview of AD
by National Institutes of Health

www.MedicalNutritionFacts.com
Free Detailed Nutrition Plans for AD,
and a Variety of Other Medical Conditions

AD Food Selection Guide: Helpful Hints for Treatment and Prevention

Do you usually start the day with cereal, instant oatmeal, or white toast? Try non-fat plain yogurt (no sugar added), berries/nuts, steal-cut oats or egg-white omelet with broccoli, spinach, and non-fat shredded cheese.

Two packets of sugar in your coffee? Try decreasing to one and a half, and then again to one packet (or less!) slowly over time so that your taste buds can accommodate. Or try minimally processed natural sweeteners, like agave nectar, a touch of honey (raw, unfiltered), or stevia (natural sugar substitute) instead.

Only have cranberry, orange, or apple juice in the refrigerator? Fill half the cup with water, add ice, and then fill the rest up with juice. Better yet, drink a full glass of water first at the start of your meal.

In the cereal aisle at the supermarket? Choose those high in fiber (greater than 6 gm/serving), which helps to slow digestion and reduce sugar/insulin level fluctuations in the blood. All-Bran® (Extra Fiber) and Kashi® (Go Lean) are two to consider.

Used to having a sandwich for lunch? Try a salad instead, adding lean turkey or grilled chicken breast, with berries, avocado, chick peas, beans, berries, flaxseeds, and a drizzle of extra virgin olive oil, fat-free balsamic, or raspberry vinaigrette.

Can't say no to bread? Say yes to 100% whole grain, containing at least a few grams of fiber per serving.

Craving french fries? Replace with oven-baked sweet potato fries.

Cheese, please? Try fat-free cheddar, swiss, cream, or cottage cheese.

Soups on? Gazpacho, miso broth, or vegetable with cubes of turkey, chicken, or tofu.

Prefer sweetened iced tea? Start by adding half as much sweetener as usual, then reduce the amount added gradually over several weeks until your taste buds accommodate. Or try minimally processed natural sweeteners, like agave nectar or a small amount of honey (raw, unfiltered) instead.

Eating a heavy dinner? Add some vinegar to your salad before the meal, which may help to delay digestion, thereby reducing glycemic index.

Dining out? Look for the health-conscious menu—most restaurants (even fast food) have several options on the menu.

Pasta night? Try spaghetti squash, or a small serving of 100% whole-grain pasta, cooked firm, which lowers glycemic index.

Think white rice is nice? How about brown rice (e.g., brown Basmati), quinoa, couscous, or barley instead.

In the mood for mashed potatoes? Try mashed cauliflower instead. Other root vegetables like celery root or turnips work too.

An alcoholic drink with dinner? A daily glass of red (or white) wine may be good for the heart and brain.

Need a snack between meals, can't say no to dessert, or no time for a full meal since you

are on the go? Try a small handful of nuts (due to fat content, should be consumed in moderation), or fruit instead, like berries (examples listed in the earlier chapters), or better yet a smoothie (with fresh fruits and vegetables, no added sugar and non-fat milk or yogurt).

Chocoholic? Small amounts of dark chocolate, low-carb, sugar-free, or sweetened with sugar alcohols may be best (e.g., mannitol, sorbitol).

APPENDIX C.
Food Terminology: An Overview

The following list will help readers understand the dietary and nutrition options available at the supermarket, health food stores, restaurants, and in their own kitchen.

Organic: Certified to be produced by certain standards (e.g., handling, storage, production) and ingredients are free from prohibited substances (e.g., synthetic pesticides, chemical fertilizers) and are not genetically modified. In the U.S., production is managed via the Organic Foods Production Act (OFPA), which integrates cultural, biological, and mechanical methods that foster "cycling of resources, promote ecological balance, and conserve biodiversity."

Enriched vs. Fortified: *Enriched* refers to replacement of lost nutrients after processing. This includes the vitamins folic acid, iron, niacin, riboflavin, and thiamine, often necessary to meet FDA standards. When making food choices, enriched foods indicate that the food has been processed, thereby losing nutrients. Avoid this type of processed food when possible, and preferentially choose fresh (or raw) food, either with or without fortified nutrients. *Fortified* refers to nutrients that are added to the food, in addition to the nutrients that were in the food originally. However, this does not necessarily make them a healthier option relative to fresh foods.

Fresh Food: No processing, preservation, or freezing. Also referred to as raw food.

"Excellent Source of," "High," "Rich in": Contains at least 20% of the Daily Value of a specific nutrient or type of dietary fiber.

Bran: The covering, or outer part of the grain, which contains the highest concentration of fiber, B vitamins, and antioxidants.

Whole Grain: Contains all of the naturally occurring elements, such as the bran, endosperm (e.g., starchy carbohydrates, protein) and germ. Whole wheat is a form of whole grain. Wheat is just one (healthy) form of grain. The important thing is to look for "whole" on the packaging (or first ingredient), and avoid "multi-grain" or "seven-grain," as these may still not contain the most healthy parts of the grains.

Extra-Virgin Olive Oil: Produced from pressing the olives without the addition of solvents. Must have low free-acidity (<0.8%), which indicates higher quality. Still high in saturated fat and calories (so use small amounts) but shown to raise HDL ("good") cholesterol.

Trans Fat: Linked to obesity, heart disease, accelerated aging, and cancer. Difficult for the body to break down. Be aware that foods that advertise having "no trans fat" may still be high in saturated (and/or unsaturated) fat and calories. In addition, FDA regulations allow food processors to write "zero trans fats" on the label even if the food actually contains 0.49 grams (per serving). If you take a look at the ingredients, you may see partially hydrogenated oil, which is the primary source of trans fat.

Saturated Fat: High intake is linked to heart disease, obesity, and some cancers. Can raise LDL cholesterol (the "bad" cholesterol). There are a number of saturated fats, some safer than others. In general, however, it is a good idea to limit saturated fats.

Polyunsaturated Fat: Contains a balance of omega-3 and omega-6 fatty acids.

Monounsaturated Fat: Sometimes called the "heart-healthy fat," which can actually reduce the "bad" cholesterol (LDL).

"Omega-3" Eggs: Hens are fed diet rich in omega-3 fatty acids (e.g., flaxseeds, alpha-linolenic acid). Look for brands with at least 200 mg per egg.

"Cage-free" Eggs: The U.S. Department of Agriculture requires only that hens spend part of its time outside in order for producers to label them as "cage-free" or "free-range" eggs. It is important to note that "cage-free" does not necessarily imply "organic." Organic eggs are from hens fed organic feed and not given antibiotics. Organic eggs are frequently higher in omega-3 fatty acids, making them a healthier option relative to regular (and most cage-free) eggs.

Egg Substitutes: Made with egg whites, which usually have 0 mg of cholesterol (¼ cup) versus over 200 mg in one equivalently sized large egg. Some brands contain up to 99% of egg whites, along with a mixture of dairy products, vegetable gums, vitamins, and other nutrients. The refrigerated Egg Beaters® Original is one example to be considered.

Glycemic Index (GI): Classification system to indicate the relative blood glucose response to carbohydrate-containing foods. It is a ranking on a scale from 0 to 100 of carbohydrates according to the extent to which they raise blood glucose levels (and subsequently, how much insulin is released by the body as a response). Low GI foods produce less of a pronounced increase in blood glucose and insulin levels, likely due to their slow metabolism, digestion, and/or absorption. High

GI foods require more insulin to metabolize and cause a more pronounced increase in blood glucose.

Sugar Substitutes: Simulate the taste of sugar, have fewer calories (energy), and can be made out of natural or synthetic components. Six are currently approved for use in the U.S. (five synthetic: aspartame, sucralose, neotame, acesulfame potassium, saccharin; one natural: stevia).

Artificial Sweeteners: Do not affect blood sugar levels but are made of synthetic compounds. At the time of publication of this book, while there is ongoing controversy over whether artificial sweeteners pose health risks, the FDA has not been presented with sufficient scientific evidence to deem them unsafe. There is, however, some evidence to suggest that beverages with artificial sweeteners may become hazardous if kept at elevated temperatures (above 80°F) for several days. Further study is indeed warranted.

High-Fructose Corn Syrup (HFCS): While having the same relative sweetness as fructose, it is highly processed and, most important, has a high glycemic index. Despite associated health concerns (e.g., obesity, metabolic syndrome), due to several reasons (e.g., lower cost than refined sugar, prolongation of shelf life, ease of mixing in beverages), HFCS use in food manufacturing has become widespread today.

Minimally Processed Natural Sweeteners: A variety of sweeteners derived from plants. Some of the more recent and popular choices include agave nectar, stevia, and raw (unfiltered) honey. Others include unsulfured blackstrap molasses, raw dried dates/date sugar, and 100% pure dark maple syrup. These types of sweeteners have somewhat of a "stronger" taste, so the same desired sweetness can be achieved by using less of it, thereby reducing caloric intake, blood glucose, and insulin release. Overuse of these sweeteners may negate their potential for benefit.

Sugar Alcohols: Also known as polyols, these are less sweet than sugar, have fewer calories, and have a lower glycemic index.

Refined Sugar: Sugar that has gone through the

process of extracting out the sugar (sucrose) from the plant materials and then removing other unwanted materials from the extracted raw sugar (e.g., stalk fibers from the sugar cane or sugar beets). Completely refined white sugar is nearly 100% sucrose and essentially contains no nutritional elements (e.g., vitamins, minerals, proteins), accounting for expressions like "empty calories" or "junk food." In the last few years, a new refined sugar with a lower GI was released in Australia. Per the company website, LoGiCane® is less refined than white, raw, and brown sugar and retains many of the nutrients usually washed out in processing (e.g., polyphenols, antioxidants, organic minerals and calcium).

APPENDIX D.
Alzheimer's Disease Research Centers

ALABAMA (AL)

University of Alabama

www.uab.edu/adc • 205-934-3847

ARIZONA (AZ)

Banner Alzheimer's Institute

www.azalz.org • 602-239-6525

ARKANSAS (AR)

University of Arkansas

alzheimer.uams.edu • 501-603-1294

CALIFORNIA (CA)

Stanford University

alzheimer.stanford.edu • 650-852-3287

University of California @ Davis
alzheimer.ucdavis.edu • 916-734-5496

University of California @ Irvine
www.alz.uci.edu • 949-824-5847

University of California @ Los Angeles
www.adc.ucla.edu • 310-206-6397

University of California @ San Diego
adrc.ucsd.edu • 858-622-5800

University of California @ San Francisco
memory.ucsf.edu • 415-476-6880

University of Southern California
www.usc.edu/dept/gero/ADRC • 213-740-7777

FLORIDA (FL)

Byrd Alzheimer's Institute
www.floridaadrc.org • 866-700-7773

GEORGIA (GA)

Emory University
www.med.emory.edu/ADC • 404-728-6950

ILLINOIS (IL)

Northwestern University
www.brain.northwestern.edu • 312-908-9339

Rush University Medical Center
www.rush.edu/radc • 312-942-2362

INDIANA (IN)

Indiana Alzheimer Disease Center
iadc.iupui.edu • 317-278-5500

KENTUCKY (KY)

University of Kentucky Alzheimer's Center
www.mc.uky.edu/coa • 859-323-6040

MARYLAND (MD)

John Hopkins University
www.alzresearch.org • 410-502-5164

MASSACHUSETTS (MA)

Boston University
www.bu.edu/alzresearch • 617-638-5368

Massachusetts General Hospital
www.madrc.org • 617-726-3987

MICHIGAN (MI)

University of Michigan
www.med.umich.edu/alzheimers • 734-764-2190

MINNESOTA (MN)

Mayo Clinic
mayoresearch.mayo.edu/mayo/research/
alzheimers_center • 507-284-1324

MISSOURI (MO)

Washington University
alzheimer.wustl.edu • 314-286-2882

NEW YORK (NY)

Columbia University
www.alzheimercenter.org • 212-305-1818

Mount Sinai School of Medicine
www.mssm.edu/psychiatry/adrc • 212-241-8329

New York University
www.med.nyu.edu/adc • 212-263-8088

NORTH CAROLINA (NC)

Duke University Medical Center
adrc.mc.duke.edu • 866-444-2372

OREGON (OR)

Oregon Health and Science University
www.ohsu.edu/research/alzheimers
503-494-6976

PENNSYLVANIA (PA)

University of Pennsylvania
www.uphs.upenn.edu/ADC
215-662-7810

University of Pittsburgh
www.adrc.pitt.edu • 412-692-2700

TEXAS (TX)

University of Texas @ Southwestern
www.utsouthwestern.edu/alzheimers/research
214-648-9376

WASHINGTON (WA)

University of Washington
www.depts.washington.edu/adrcweb
206-277-3281

For an updated list of the Alzheimer's Disease Research Centers located in the U.S., please visit the NIH website: www.nia.nih.gov/Alzheimers/ Research Information/ResearchCenters.

On this site, there is a document that can be downloaded with a full Alzheimer's Disease Center Directory. The detailed directory includes comprehensive information such as contact names and the full addresses of each of the centers.

Brain-Healthy Menu Options

EXAMPLE DAILY MENUS FOR BRAIN-HEALTHY EATING

MONDAY	
Breakfast	Scrambled eggs. 3 egg whites or egg substitute, scrambled in a little skim milk, with chopped fresh tomato, onion, and spinach. Serve with 1 slice rye toast. Black or green tea or coffee.
Lunch	Tuna or chicken lettuce wrap. Mix tuna or chunked chicken with fat-free mayonnaise and raisins. Wrap in full piece lettuce.
Snack	Chips and salsa dip. Flaxseed tortilla chips. Mix $1/2$ cup salsa with fresh avocado and 1 tbsp fat-free sour cream.
Dinner	Flatbread pepperoni pizza. 1 glass Concord grape juice.
Dessert	Cinnamon baked apples. Sliced apples baked with cinnamon, small amount raw honey, topped with Kashi GoLean Crunch.

TUESDAY	
Breakfast	Pancakes. Whole-wheat or flaxseed pancakes sweetened with sucralose and/or applesauce (no sugar added). Add blueberries, raspberries, and strawberries. Use cooking spray on the pan. Up to 2 tbsp maple syrup if desired. Black or green tea or coffee.
Lunch	Boca burger.
Snack	Trail mix with peanuts, almonds, raisins, and dried apricots.

| Dinner | Chicken with balsamic fig sauce. 1 glass Concord grape juice. |
| Dessert | Cupcakes. Make with steel-cut oats, peanut butter, blueberries, protein or cocoa powder, and sugar-free sweetener. |

WEDNESDAY	
Breakfast	Egg-white western omelet. 3 egg whites or egg substitute with fat free cheese and spinach, topped with salsa, and made with cooking spray. One-third cup black or baked beans. Black or green tea or coffee.
Lunch	Tuna and soup. Half tuna-salad sandwich made with fat-free mayonnaise on 1 slice rye toast. Bowl of low-sodium chicken, vegetable, lentil or split-pea soup.
Snack	Hummus with raw vegetables, such as carrots, broccoli, and cauliflower.
Dinner	Herbed steak. 1 glass red wine.
Dessert	Hot fudge sundae.

THURSDAY	
Breakfast	Fruit smoothie. Blend $1/2$ cup strawberries and blueberries with $1/2$ cup Greek yogurt and $1/3$ cup ice. Add 2 tsp sugar-free sweetener. Black or green tea or coffee.
Lunch	Spinach salad. Fresh spinach with chunks of chicken, walnuts, and pomegranate seeds. Fat-free balsamic vinaigrette dressing.
Snack	Protein bar (see Chapter 6 for optimum brain-healthy criteria).
Dinner	Grilled rosemary salmon skewers. 1 glass Concord grape juice.
Dessert	Strawberries 'n cream. Chopped strawberries with $1/2$ cup fat-free half and half. Add small amount sucralose to desired sweetness.

FRIDAY	
Breakfast	Poached egg with barley and spinach. Black or green tea or coffee.
Lunch	Moo shu chicken.
Snack	Large apple and $1/2$ cup pumpkin seeds.
Dinner	Antipasto. Whole-wheat pasta with chopped broccoli, carrots, zucchini, and arugula. Add 2 tbsp extra virgin olive oil, 2 tbsp balsamic vinegar, 2 tbsp cooking wine, and $1/4$ cup grated parmesan cheese. 1 glass red wine.
Dessert	Fruit, nut, and chocolate cup. Top 1 cup blueberries, raspberries, and strawberries with 1 tablespoon dark-chocolate chips and 1 tablespoon chopped nuts.

SATURDAY	
Breakfast	Oatmeal. Rolled oat oatmeal with blueberries, sugar-free sweetener. Black or green tea or coffee.
Lunch	Citrus-chili shrimp.
Snack	Fruit salad and nuts. 1 cup fruit salad. $1/3$ cup of dry roasted almonds, hazelnuts, walnuts, pecans, pistachios, cashews, or macadamia nuts.
Dinner	Grilled salmon. Large grilled salmon steak topped with 2 tbsp mango salsa, served with asparagus and $1/3$ cup whole grain brown rice. 1 glass red wine.
Dessert	Chocolate indulgence. 2 oz 90-percent cocoa dark chocolate (approximately $1/2$ bar). 1 cup skim milk with cocoa powder.

SUNDAY	
Breakfast	Berry and flaxseed breakfast smoothie. Black or green tea or coffee.
Lunch	Lentil soup. Low-sodium lentil soup with $1/2$ cup chunks of chicken or ham added. 1 slice rye toast.
Snack	Peanut butter muffin. Spread 1 tbsp natural no-sugar-added peanut butter on whole-grain toast or English muffin.
Dinner	Curry chicken. Prepare with extra virgin olive oil. Serve with whole-grain brown rice. 1 glass Concord grape juice.
Dessert	Sundae Top. 3 tbsp fat-free whip cream with $1/2$ cup raspberries and blackberries on top. Add $1/4$ cup nuts if desired.

GENERAL GUIDELINES FOR BRAIN-HEALTHY DIET (PERCENT DAILY INTAKE):

Include the following suggested breakdown of macronutrients (modified from Craft study):

- Fat: 25 percent (less than 7 percent of which saturated)
- Carbohydrates: 30–45 percent (low-glycemic index)
- Protein: 25–35 percent

Index

treatment. *see also*
  comprehensive treatment;
  multimodal therapy
  overview, 3–5, 13–19
  drugs, 51–59
  not recommended by
    author, 135–136
  patient-centered care, 14–19,
    35–37
  prescription drugs, 3
  strategies, 33, 37–38
  20-Step Plan, 142–150
treatment and prevention
  strategy combination,
  37–38
turmeric root (curcumin), 65,
  70–71, 134, 146, 172–173,
  222
20-Step Plan for Alzheimer's
  Treatment, 142–150

unsaturated fats, 89, 106, 199

vaccine treatment, 127, 142
Valium (diazepam), 121
Valproic Acid (divalproex),
  119
vascular dementia, 162, 218

vascular risk factors, 112, 148,
  158–160, 162, 218,
  221–222. *see also* high
  blood pressure
vegetables, 92, 190
very low-carbohydrate diets,
  105, 110–111, 205–211
video games, 80, 147, 178, 221
visiting nurses, 124
vitamin B_6, 174, 202, 206
vitamin B_{12}, 103, 173, 174,
  203, 222
vitamin D, 103, 149, 173, 202,
  222
vitamin E, 135
vitamins. *see specific vitamins;*
  supplements

weight training, 79, 176
Western diet, 11, 94, 154–155,
  191
"white matter hyperintensities,"
  159
whole grain, 234–235
worry, 214–215
Wright, C.B., 159

Zoloft (sertraline), 116–117
zolpidem (Ambien), 121

Notes

Notes

Notes

Notes